P9-ARE-708

FINE
beauty

FINE
beauty

Beauty Basics and Beyond for African-American Women

SAM FINE

with Julia Chance

Riverhead Books
New York
1998

CREATIVE DIRECTOR LLOYD BOSTON
ART DIRECTOR CLAIRE VACCARO
DESIGNER RENATO STANISIC

Julia Chance is the associate fashion and beauty editor at *Essence*
magazine. Her firsthand knowledge of the unique beauty needs and
desires of African-American women has helped give a comprehensible
voice to this project.

A native of Baltimore, Julia graduated from Hampton Institute.
She lives in Brooklyn, New York.

RIVERHEAD BOOKS
a member of
Penguin Putnam Inc.
200 Madison Avenue
New York, NY 10016

Library of Congress Cataloging-in-Publication Data

Fine, Sam.
    Fine beauty : beauty basics and beyond for African-American women/
    by Sam Fine.
        p. cm.
    ISBN 1-57322-095-7
    1. Beauty, Personal. 2. Afro-American women. 3. Cosmetics.
    I. Title.
    RA778.4.A36F56   1998   97-38059 CIP
    646.7'042'08996073—dc21

Printed in the United States of America
10 9 8 7 6 5 4 3 2 1
This book is printed on acid-free paper. ∞

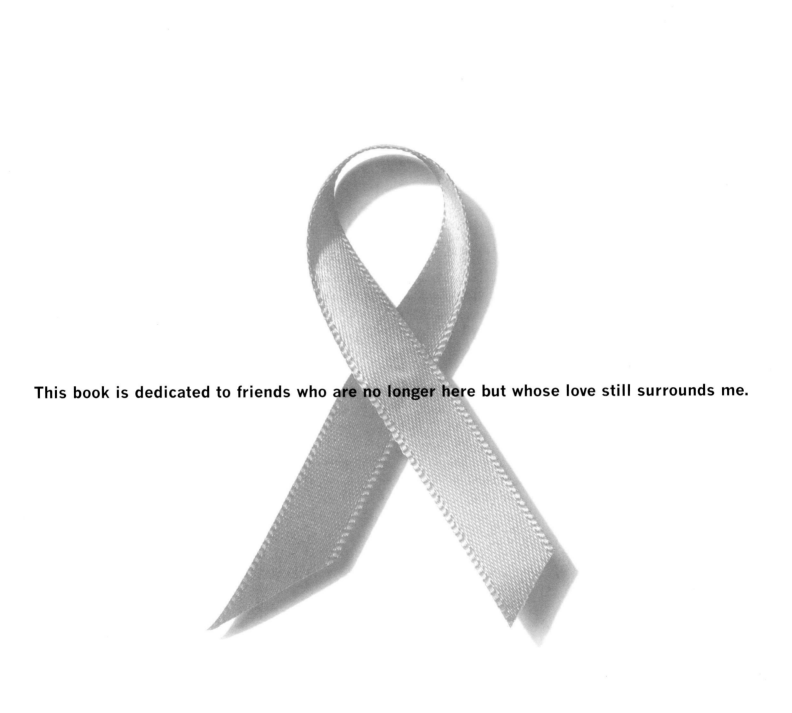

This book is dedicated to friends who are no longer here but whose love still surrounds me.

A portion of the proceeds from this book will be donated to God's Love We Deliver.

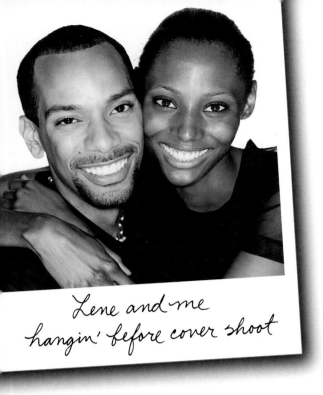

Lene and me hangin' before cover shoot

CONTENTS

THE OTHER DAY
ME HOW I LEARNED
PERFECTLY. THE ANSWER

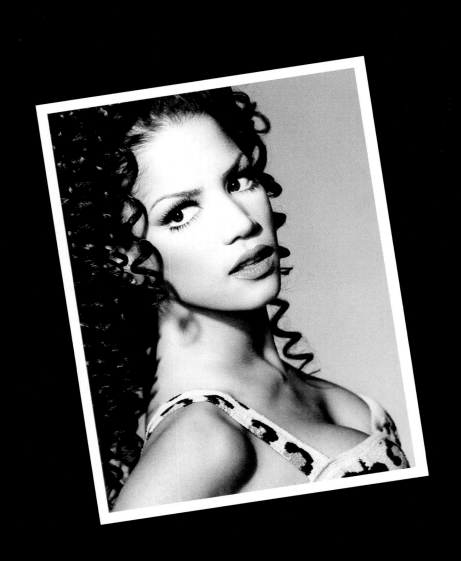

MY BOYFRIEND ASKED TO DO MY MAKEUP WAS SIMPLE: SAM FINE.

But Sam wasn't always around. . . . When my mother broke the news to me at thirteen that it was time for me to become "refined" (code word for making the transition from kid to lady), the lessons did not include using makeup. Momma's from a generation of women who didn't experiment with makeup in their teens and twenties, because nothing was available for them. For my sisters and me growing up in Detroit, the only examples of glamorized black women were Diana Ross and disco queens like Patti LaBelle, Chaka Khan, and Donna Summer. It was hard to find more natural-looking images of models and celebrities whose makeup I could copy, and I was frustrated at the lack of range between an everyday look and the roar of the greasepaint. But it didn't stop me from trying. I'd go to the drugstore after school and gleefully toss my baby-sitting money over the counter for some beauty basics like a compact, a bottle of foundation, blush, and eye shadow. I'd take the magic potions home thinking I'd apply them and get a head-turning effect. Boy, did I! At school everyone noticed me—because my make-up was so horrible!

I had no idea how to choose or apply foundation. I'd be smiling through a thick pink mask that didn't blend into my hairline or over my jaw. The blush was too bright, the eye shadow migrated across my temples like rain clouds, and my idea of what to do with eyeliner would have won me an Oscar if I'd played a villain in a Batman flick. It didn't take long before hazing by the boys in the class (and messages from my mother and her friends that I looked ridiculous, relayed to me through other kids) got to me, and I gave up.

Years later I became a model. I thought that once I got into the business I would learn how to do a professional job on my face in no time. Every modeling career starts out the same: You learn how to model by doing "test shots" with a photographer. Basically it's two amateurs getting together and trying to re-create what they've seen in magazines. When you're testing you have to bring the clothes yourself and do your own hair and makeup. I did the best I could and felt pretty confident on that long-ago day in 1984 when I stepped onto seamless paper under the photographer's bright lights. But when the pictures came back I was shattered by what I saw—every single mistake I'd made trying to put my look together was magnified a thousand times. I continued to test and do my early bookings for magazines like *Seventeen,* but what was required in terms of hair and makeup remained foreign to me. I never imagined that I'd have to sit for an hour to have my makeup done, or that it would take so many specific steps (concealer, pressed powder, loose powder, and so on) to get an "ideal" result. And I certainly didn't expect that a professional makeup artist would be just as confounded as I was in addressing the needs of African-American beauty, especially when it came to matching foundations and powders to my skin tone. More often than not, the person paid to do the makeup would ask me if I had my own foundation, a question I've almost never heard posed to my white counterparts. Sometimes I'd get lucky and a seasoned pro would pull out a palette like something a painter would have, and spend ten minutes mixing the colors for my face. I would always be grateful for the diligence, but it was disheartening, because it wasn't something I had the money or the eye to repeat on my own.

Sometime in 1990, Fran Cooper, a hugely successful black make-up artist, had the grace to tell all of us black girls peddling polyester on the runways to look out for "the kid from Chicago with the ponytail," who could "paint on a dime." Fran was talking about Sam Fine, who'd come to New York City to try his luck with his paints and brushes.

The first time I spotted Sam, he was one of ten assistants working under the head makeup artist at an Isaac Mizrahi fashion show. Sam was a tender twenty-one, excited and smiling like it was his first day of school. In the hierarchy of the fashion business Sam was then a nobody. But because there were, and are, so few black faces behind the scenes in the fashion business, I wanted to take a leap of faith and help a brother out. I started ordering him around like a moving man, telling him where to put each stroke of color and which brush-es to use to get the shadows just right. Little did I know he was way ahead of me. I was the one getting schooled. "I've had my worst fear come true a lot, when I try to help somebody out," I told him, "and it's that you'll screw me up so bad I'll look like the victim of a hate crime." Sam laughed and painted away with complete confidence. We both had plenty to be nervous about. The look Mizrahi wanted for the show was a seventies makeup extravaganza. All the models were supposed to get painted like an old Grace Jones album cover, with parrot-wing eye shadow and eyebrows plucked near as bald as a broiler chicken. It wasn't an obvious thing to pull off, and if Sam or I couldn't do it, neither one of us would have a job. I started to relax, release, and relate, though, because I could tell he was transforming me into the best version of myself. An hour later, when I looked in the mirror, I was impressed by his work. From that moment I knew that Sam and I had a future. And what a future it would be!

It began with Sam's tweezing my brows, and escalated to my entrusting him to do everything. He would be right there with me, giving instructions to the hairdresser on how to cut and highlight my hair or calling Versace to order my evening gowns for a major event. Sam's work was indispensable. He was one-stop shopping, a full-service salon on two feet. He went above and beyond the call of duty; he had to see what he called his "vision" come to life.

It wasn't long before word of mouth spread about Sam, and I didn't have him all to myself. I may not have had him with me all the time anymore, but he left me armed with the skills to protect myself when I was on shoots with someone who was just starting to know my face. And I was no longer dominated by the makeup kit, each product an unruly youngster running all over me the minute I let it out. Sam taught me how to use makeup properly and how not to be afraid of it. Once we got that down, I had the self-confidence and the room to play.

In the spring of 1994, I made fashion history by being the first African-American to be awarded a cosmetics contract with Revlon. I had gotten through the door, and I wanted Sam to come with me. My contract stipulated that I had my choice of makeup artist, but sadly, in modeling, as in every other area of business, the top level is often closed to black hair and makeup artists. The higher you go, the fewer black faces you see. Still, I knew I had to have Sam with me. The first ad campaign I worked on was done with talented people chosen by the company. While those pictures turned out fine, my feeling of triumph was undercut by the fact that the team wasn't African-American. On the next round of shootings I was blessed to have my people with me. It was great to be there after ten years of working as a model, and to see myself the way I had imagined looking throughout my entire career. But my vanity aside, it made me really proud that when I got Sam through the door, he didn't come just to look around—he started rearranging the furniture! The next thing I knew, Sam was a Revlon spokesperson. And the professional help I was getting from him was available to the sister next door.

Every woman, whether she's a professional model, a homemaker, a doctor, or a factory worker, wants to see herself at her best. We all see ourselves as beautiful in one of two ways: natural or glamorous. But we need education and guidance to help us achieve our ideals. Having the skills to do your makeup properly saves you from the tyranny of being dictated to or discouraged by fashion, or making mistakes that can be costly in terms of time and money. Working with Sam, I've learned how to throw my face together in five minutes, or spend time getting ready for a glitzy gala with equal skill. Every time someone notices my makeup now and says, "You look great," I smile secretly. Because when I say, "Thanks," I know I'm really thanking Sam.

—Veronica Webb

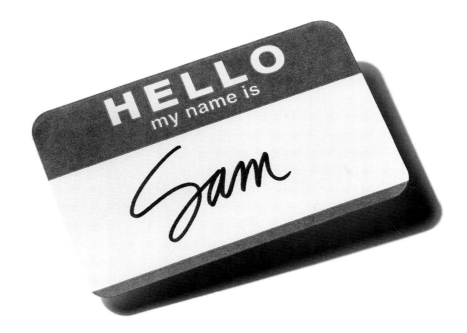

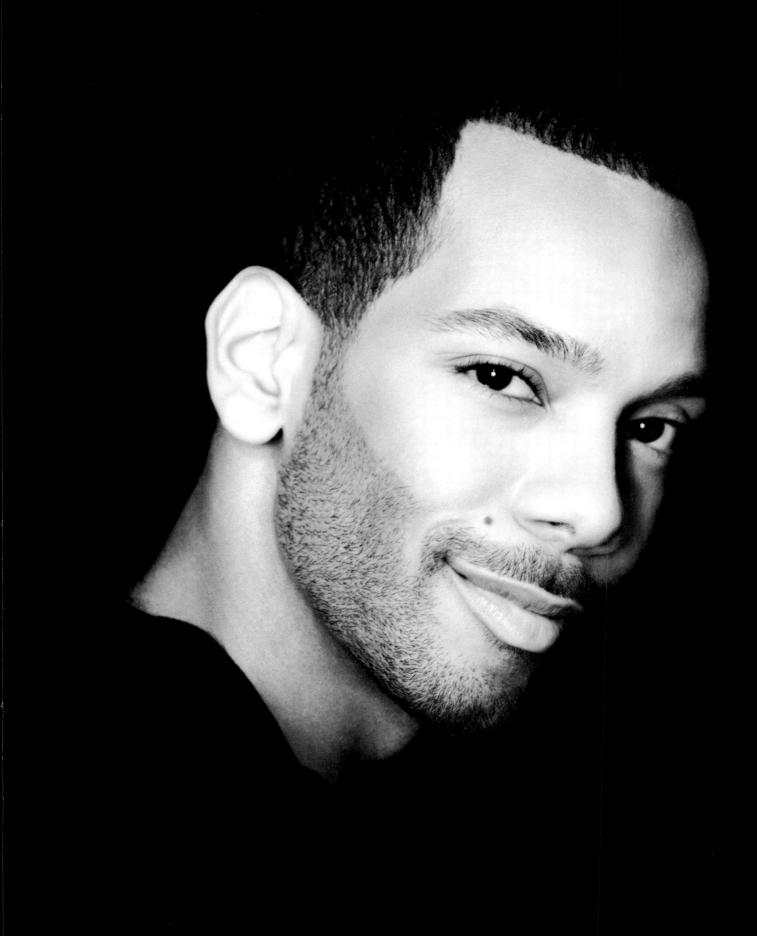

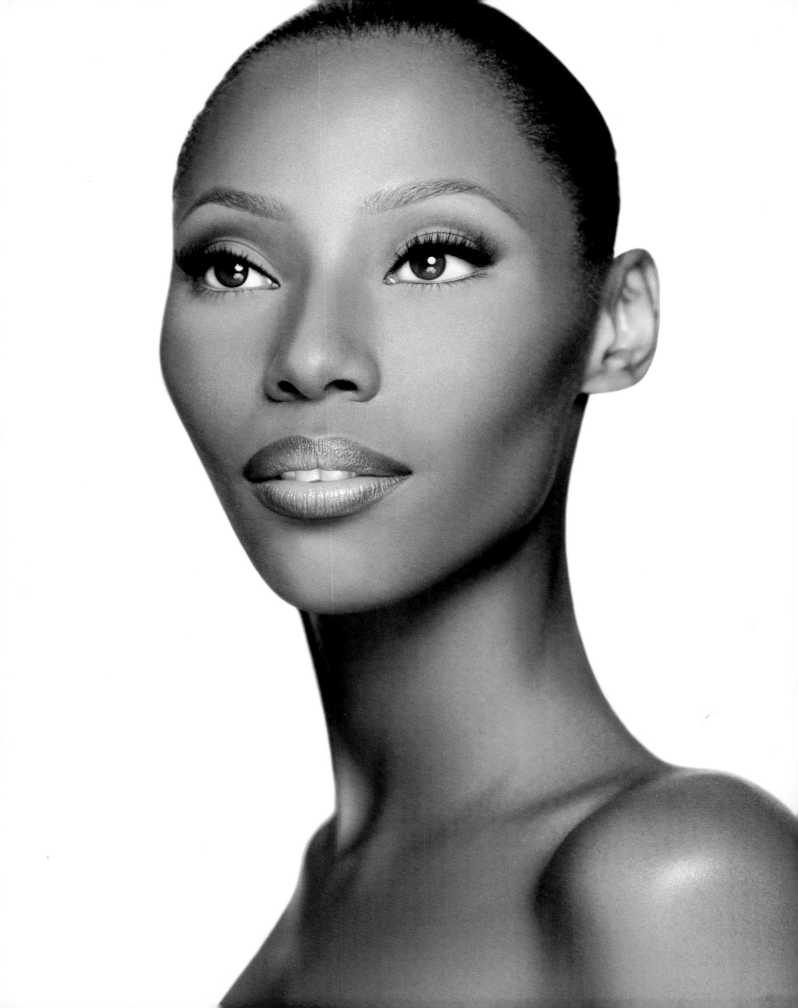

MY TAKE ON MAKEUP

My first brush with makeup occurred when, as a boy, I watched my mother apply it. Her beauty regime consisted of applying base and powder and grooming her eyebrows. To do anything more, to her, would have seemed too much. Like many African-American women of her generation, she couldn't envision herself being as glamorous as the prevailing beauty icons. At a time when women such as Marilyn Monroe or Jackie Kennedy were society's standards of beauty, she was hard-pressed to find self-affirming images to fashion herself after. And with the exception of Lena Horne, or later Diahann Carroll, African-American beauty icons were few and far between. Also, along with their not having beauty icons to associate with, there was a limited amount of makeup suitable for African-American women. Makeup colors that were available did not always compliment their complexions, and special formulations for women of color were unheard of. No wonder Mom kept it simple.

Today much of that has changed. African-American women are embracing their beauty as never before. From the scintillating sizzle of Tyra Banks and the urban chic of Mary J. Blige to the sophisticated glamour of Vanessa Williams and the ageless allure of Patti LaBelle, sisters are finally getting to see just how glamorous they can be. Not since the "Look, Ma! There's colored people on television!" days in the late sixties and early seventies—when Diana Ross and the Supremes topped the music charts, Lola Falana shimmied and high-kicked on *The Flip Wilson Show,* and Pam Grier gave us a taste of just how "Foxy" she could be—have we been privy to such a variety of black beauty on parade. And in recent years, the "browning of America" has led cosmetics manufacturers to make and market products with the specific needs of African-American women in mind, thus enabling them to feel more confident about finding cosmetics to suit them. But when you consider the fact that the first African-American with a major cosmetics contract was not signed up until 1994, or that the appearance of a black face on the cover of top fashion magazines is still an event, you realize that we have a ways to go.

Beauty role models and the right shades of makeup are great, but you also need information that's geared toward you. *That's* what's been lacking. Working with Mikki Taylor one day and Naomi Campbell the next confirmed for me what I already sensed: Black women have special needs. In searching for themselves in most mainstream makeup guides, if they are addressed at all, they often find guidance limited to just a few vague general tips, usually with one or two models shown to represent all black women. Worse yet, the tone of those guides can be unaffirming, with an attitude that's more about correcting what's "wrong" than about appreciating an African-American woman's unique beauty.

Long before I shaped the brows of Veronica Webb, applied false eyelashes to Iman, or powdered the face of Nancy Wilson, I worked behind a department store cosmetics counter, a place I consider the "real school of beauty." It was common practice there to recommend pink and coral colors to sisters with light complexions, while darker sisters were usually relegated to plums and reds. Black women had for so long been programmed to believe they needed these colors to make their complexions come alive that when a more nude trend in makeup began—fleshy beiges, rosy nudes, and other neutrals— sisters could not envision themselves in such colors. I made it my mission to show African-American women how to break out of this color-coded approach and persuaded them to try shades that would play up their natural coloring. From then on, every woman who visit- ed my counter found herself leaving with a neutral palette, and a new appreciation for her beauty. Neutral became my mantra, and in no time we were selling out of anything that came close to a natural shade. It wasn't long before I took all that I'd learned from the real school of beauty and began using it on free-lance jobs. You should have seen the look on Patti LaBelle's face when, after she had worn bright red lipstick for years, I suggested she try a tawny brown shade with a hint of gold in the middle. Now *she* insists on wearing neutral shades, not only in lip color but in blushers and eye shadows too.

My take on beauty is simple: Makeup should be fun. It's not brain surgery, so don't overthink it. Instead, explore the many beau- tiful possibilities makeup can bring. Toss out all those rules you might've picked up on your cosmetics journey. Beauty is not about conforming to unrealistic ideals, but about finding what works for *you*. It is in this spirit that I want you to use this book. I hope it will prompt you to indulge in a new shade of lipstick, motivate you to try eye shadow for the first time, or simply allow you to feel more confident about applying makeup. Most of all, I hope it will inspire you to accept the skin you're in. You can't look to makeup to make you over. True self-satisfaction comes from within, and *that's* where your makeup regime should begin.

"SAM'S GENIUS TO BLEND MAKEUP ELEGANCE, ALWAYS DRAMATIC YET

LIES IN HIS ABILITY
BEAUTIFULLY WITH
CREATING THE MOST
NATURAL FACE."

IMAN

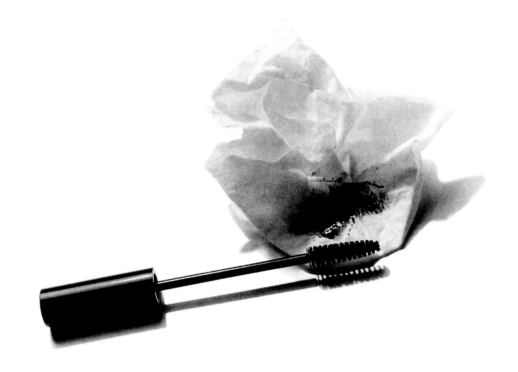

MAKEUP 101

TOOLS

Just as important as the makeup you wear are the tools you use to apply it. Look for durable sponges that won't crumble, and brushes that'll hold up to any eye shadow. Invest in good brushes, sable, fox, or pony, for instance. With proper care, including washing at least once a month in a mild detergent, they should last a lifetime. On the following pages are the tools found in my makeup bag; choose yours according to your makeup needs.

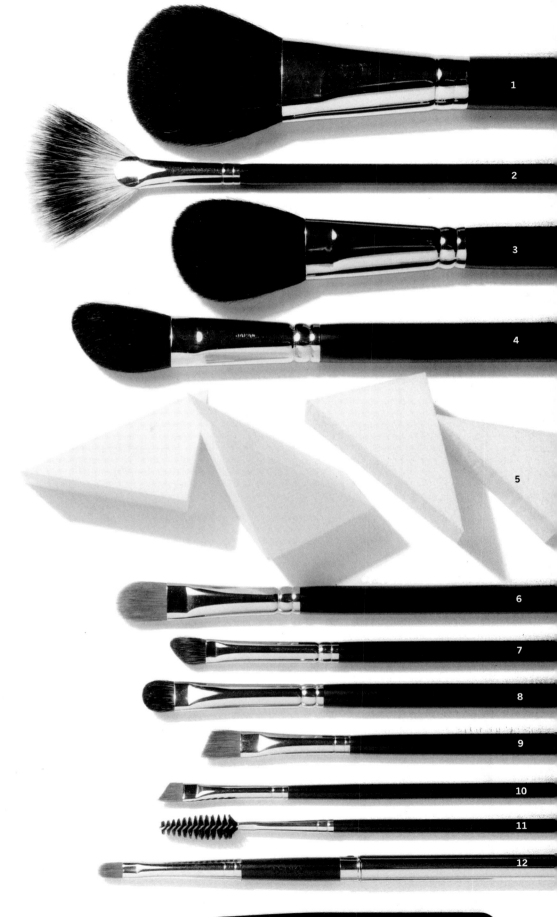

1

2

3

4

5

6

7

8

9

10

11

12

13

1. POWDER BRUSH

This comes in quite handy. It's most commonly used with loose powder to set foundation, and it can also be a blending tool to tone down and soften makeup if you feel you've gone too far.

2. WHISK BRUSH

This makeup artist's must-have sweeps away excess powder under the eyes, as well as any eye shadow fallout.

3. BLUSH BRUSH

A good one of these enables you to apply and blend blush evenly—something you couldn't possibly achieve with the miniature versions found in compacts.

4. CONTOUR BRUSH

This slightly rounded, slanted brush is great for defining cheeks and nose. Its medium size ensures soft, blended results.

5. SPONGES

The best thing going for applying and blending foundation evenly. Wedge sponges are especially good for such hard-to-reach areas as under the eyes and around the nose.

6. EYE SHADOW BRUSH

Use this brush to apply highlighter along the brow bone, to make it appear more prominent and enhance the arch of the brow.

7. EYE SHADOW BRUSH

This slanted brush is just the thing for precise application. It makes defining areas like the crease of the eye a breeze.

8. EYE SHADOW BRUSH

This fuller-size brush is great for applying shadows over the entire lid. It can also be used for blending and for softening harsh shadow lines.

9. EYELINER BRUSH

This slanted, stiff-bristled brush is great for lining top and bottom lids. It can provide a smoky line when paired with eye shadow, or a sharper, more precise line when dampened and used with cake liners.

10. EYEBROW BRUSH

Used to fill in sparse areas of the brow, this brush is my favorite for creating a fierce eyebrow.

11. EYEBROW GROOMER

In addition to keeping eyebrow hair in place, this brush makes it easier to see which hairs need to be removed by tweezing.

12. LIP BRUSH

Though it's faster to apply lipstick straight from the tube, there's nothing like the controlled application of a lip brush.

13. TWEEZERS

You can't beat the precision you get with tweezers. Razors and hair clippers may help shape the brow, but with them you're sure to have unsightly stubble in just a few days. Tweezers are by far the best tool for neatly and completely removing brow hairs.

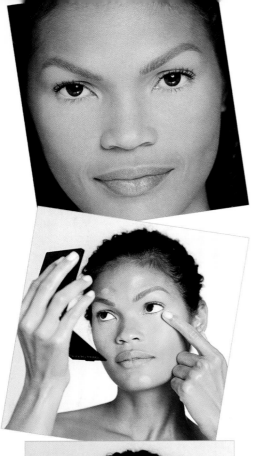

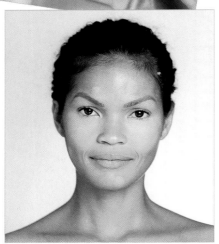

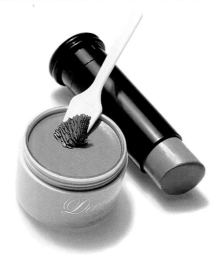

What is a concealer, and how do I use it?

Using a concealer is the first step in creating a flawless finish. Concealers cover blemishes, minor scarring, dark areas, and other imperfections and help even out the complexion. They are available in various forms—tubes, wands, pots, and sticks. I recommend those that come in a pot or a stick; they provide better coverage and are easier to regulate, whether you're going for sheer or full coverage. Concealers come in three or four shades, and you might think you have to match one to your skin like a foundation. Not true. Concealers are not supposed to be your exact color. In fact, a concealer should be one shade lighter than your natural color, in order to lighten those dark areas you want to even out. Got it? Now finish by using foundation to even out your entire complexion, then set with powder.

May I use a concealer without using foundation?

No. If you've been using concealer alone, dotting it on in certain areas, then attempting to blend it in, shame on you! That's a sure way to have raccoon eyes (light rings around the eyes). If you're looking for light coverage, use a cream formula base that is close to your color, and dab it on the areas you feel need a little help. This will give you the subtle coverage you crave, without the blotchiness you'd have with concealer alone.

CONCEALER

How do I avoid cakey-looking concealer?

Cakiness usually occurs when concealer is applied too heavily and not blended well. When applying concealer, start by scooping a small amount out of the container and allowing it to warm up on the back of your hand. This will make it glide on more smoothly. Keep in mind that the skin under the eyes is naturally thinner and less resilient, and thus more prone to cakiness, than any other part of the face. When you're applying powder here, be sure to use a light hand. For a smooth and creaseless finish, remove any excess with a small powder brush.

How do I choose the right foundation?

Foundations come in many different forms and provide many different finishes. Choosing the correct one can make your whole look, so read this carefully. Liquid foundations offer the lightest coverage, and provide a natural look. They're available in water- and oil-based formulas, so it's easy for anybody, regardless of skin type, to find the right one. Cream foundations, usually found in compacts and sticks, give the fullest coverage and the most flawless of finishes. Cream-to-powder formulas, on the other hand, allow you to experience the best of both worlds, with the look of a cream and the silky finish of a powder. Since all cream formulas contain some level of oil, if you have oily skin these might not be for you. Remember, selecting the right foundation is a result of trial and error, so don't think that if it's not right the first time it'll never work.

FOUNDATION

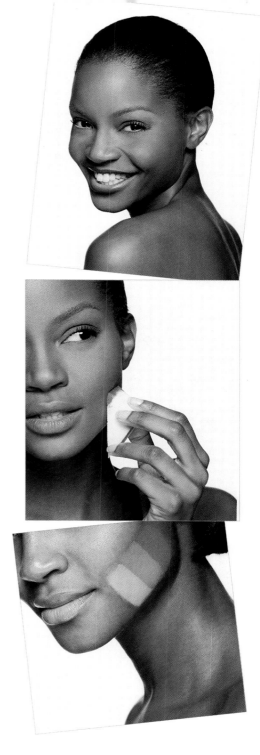

How can I find the right color?

When shopping for foundation, start by selecting three shades that are close to your complexion. Test all three for trueness by applying them to your jawline *only*—not your hand, and *definitely* not the inside of your wrist. The outer perimeter of your face (hairline, jawline) is the truest in color to the rest of your body. It is this part of your face that foundation needs to blend with easily, unless you plan to paint your whole body. Then go out into the daylight and see which of the three blends best. While you're out there, make sure the color you've chosen isn't too red or yellow for your complexion.

What's the best way to apply foundation?

Achieving beautiful-looking skin is not as simple as selecting the right base. Proper application guarantees great results. It's important to start with a good moisturizer, to ensure smooth, even coverage. (If your skin is oily, do not skip this step; simply use an oil-free moisturizer.) For quick yet flawless coverage, apply foundation with a wedge sponge. This lets you get to hard-to-reach areas around the nose and under the eyes. For the sheerest of applications, dampen your sponge. This trick helps thin the foundation, so it can glide on better.

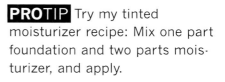

PROTIP Try my tinted moisturizer recipe: Mix one part foundation and two parts moisturizer, and apply.

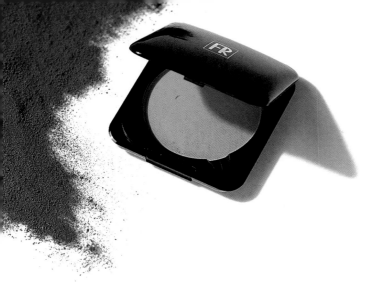

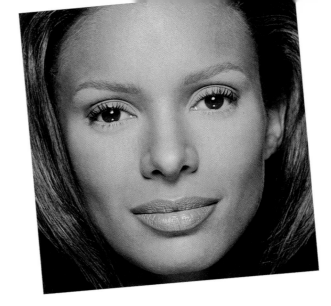

What's the purpose of powder?

Just as a top coat protects and maintains nail polish, powder sets and maintains the color and finish of your foundation. Loose powder is best for setting all foundations, except, of course, the cream-to-powder type. This type does not need powder, because it dries down to a powdery finish. Pressed powders are great for touching up oily areas such as nose and chin, and are fabulous for on-the-go touch-ups. With powders, as with foundations, it's important to choose a color as close to your natural complexion as possible. There's nothing worse than putting on the right foundation, then ruining it with a powder that's ashy or too red.

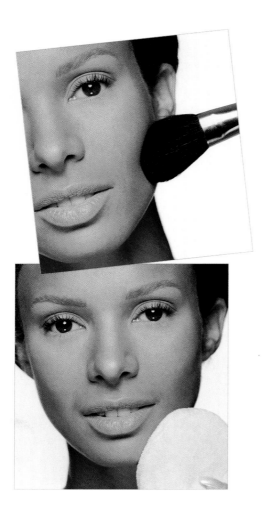

How do I combat my midday shine?

You may, like many women of color, have oily skin. While this means you'll probably stay young-looking longer than other women, you'll still want to control the situation. One way is to pull out your trusty pressed powder. Start by blotting the oily areas with a tissue to remove excess oil. then powder with a puff. Disposable blotting sheets are also great items to have on hand. These little squares of powdered paper really do the job, and with them you'll always be armed and ready.

POWDER

How do you apply powder properly?

No one can mistake you for the "walking dead" if your powder is applied correctly. So follow this simple advice: Take your trusty powder brush and pick up loose powder. Release any excess with a simple flick of the wrist. Apply liberally all over your face. Remember, your face is supposed to look drier than it would with no powder at all. If you feel you've applied too much, dampen your sponge and blot, or just give yourself a few minutes to let your natural glow come through.

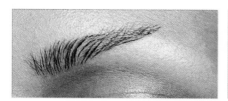
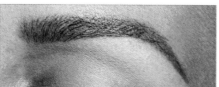
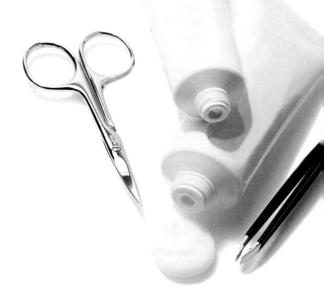

I've tweezed my eyebrows so much over the years that they don't grow back. Help!

Unfortunately, eyebrows don't grow perfectly or completely. And if you've followed the trends, you might not have any. So here's where you become an artist. Use a pencil or powder to create the desired shape. Pencils offer great control, but because they are waxy, they can appear shiny. If this happens, dust loose powder over the pencil line. Or use an angled brush, along with an eye shadow a shade lighter than your eyebrow, to fill thin areas. And remember, practice makes perfect.

EYEBROWS

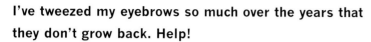
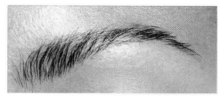
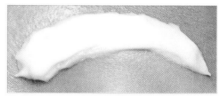
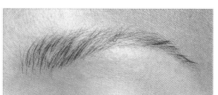

What's the point of bleaching my brows?

Lightening the brows is a great way to bring more attention to the eyes. Begin with a simple bleaching cream, which can be used to lighten facial hair as well. Mix the cream according to
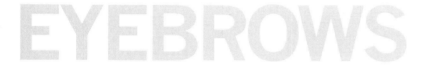
package instructions, and leave it on the brow for a minute or two, checking to make sure you're achieving the desired color. Bleaching can give you a color that ranges from warm chestnut to reddish blond. If you find that you've made your brows lighter than intended, you can always darken them with a powder or pencil.

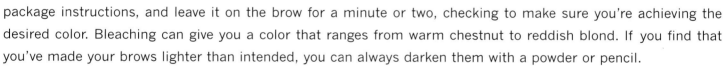
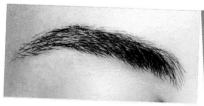
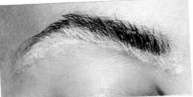
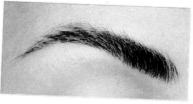

How do I find the right shape for my eyebrows?

Eyebrow shapes are like skirt lengths: they change with fashion. Unless you're the trendy type, I wouldn't recommend that you look to fashion for your brow shape. Instead, think about whether you want a stylish brow with a high arch, or one that's just well-groomed and natural. One way to find your desired shape is to draw over the hairs you don't want with a white eyeliner pencil, then tweeze. This allows you to see the brow you're going to have, and won't overdo it.

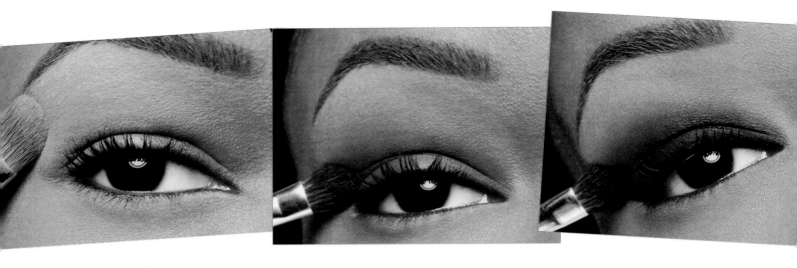

I want to use eye shadow but don't know where to begin.

There are three basic steps to apply eye shadow. The simplest is to use a natural-colored eye shadow over the entire eyelid. If you desire more definition, add a darker shadow either in the crease of the eye or from the lash line up past the crease. If drama is what you're looking for, layer farther with your darkest shadow over the same areas. For best results, don't forget to blend.

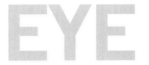

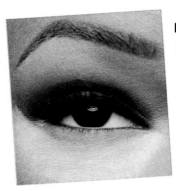

How can I prevent eye shadow from falling under my eyes?

Relax. Even the most seasoned pros have to contend with this minor inconvenience. Here's a quick and easy remedy I refer to as "fallout security." Apply loose powder directly under the eye area; this way, if eye shadow falls, it never has the chance to settle. After you've finished applying eye shadow, whisk away fallout and excess powder with a powder brush.

PROTIP Shimmer shadows are great for adding a dramatic spark to any makeup look. Place them on the browbone, the crest of the cheeks, or along the collarbone and shoulders for a luminous finish.

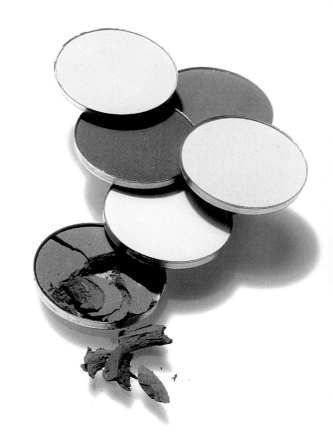

What colors should I use?

Stick with natural, brown-based shadows. Not only do they compliment any coloring, but they also leave very little room for error. When you feel more comfortable with these shades, and your ability to apply them, you may become more adventurous and try other colors. Make sure they are the right ones

SHADOW

for you, though. Maybe the blue for you is not the electric blue your fairer-skinned girlfriend wears, but a strong navy or dark gray. Keep in mind that your face is not a blank canvas. Whatever color you use will change a bit, depending on your natural coloring, and that's fine, as long as the color compliments you.

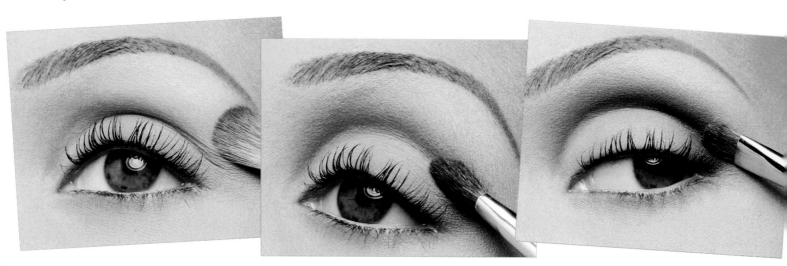

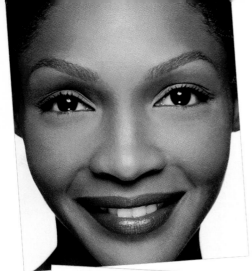

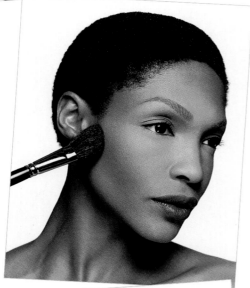

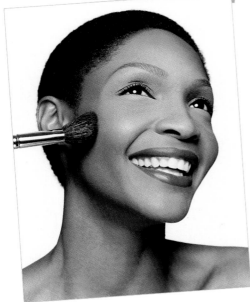

How can I find a natural-colored blush?

The notion of blush for African-American women differs from that for other women. Most black women—men too—don't blush or flush in the rosy, red-cheeked way that traditional blushers suggest. What you want to achieve with blush is a warm, natural glow. It's best to go with colors in the range from tangerine to brick red, as these echo your natural skin tone. If you want more vibrant color, use a pressed powder one shade darker than your natural color and layer your favorite color over it.

BLUSH

What's the best way to apply blush?

This is an age-old question, and everyone has a different answer, so let me set the record straight. The best way to apply blush is to start at the ear and end at the apple of the cheek. Never start at the apple of your cheek, because too much color will settle there (think circus clown). By starting at the ear, you contour as you bring color into the face. Finish with a dusting of loose powder for an even more natural look. This trick also comes in handy if you overdo it.

PROTIP Using a bronzing powder in place of blush adds warmth without introducing color.

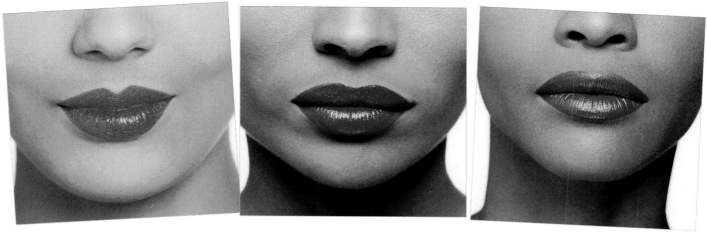

How do I pick the right shade of lipstick?

You can always be a winner in the game of lip color, if you keep in mind a simple rule: Colors come in many varieties. Take, for example, the color red. Not only are there lighter and darker shades of red, but there are also brown tones, pink tones, orange tones, and so on. The key is to test three shades of the same color, to determine which lipstick looks best on you.

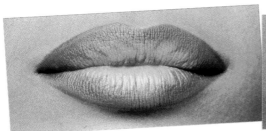 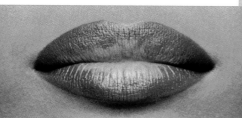 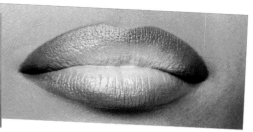

If I use a neutral lipstick, won't it look boring?

No. Neutral does not equal boring. There is a wide variety of neutral colors, ranging from rosy beiges to walnut browns to deep mochas, that look stunning on women of color. The trick to pulling it off is in defining the shape of the mouth with a lip pencil. You don't want an obvious line, so don't even *think* about pulling out that black eyeliner to rim your lips. Any number of brown pencils will do the job, without the harshness. In fact, lip liner adds definition to the mouth regardless of what shade of lipstick you're wearing. So remember, if it screams liner 'n' lipstick, chances are it needs to be blended.

LIPSTICK

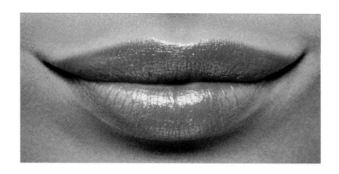

If I don't want to use liner and lipstick every day, what are my alternatives?

Try lip sheers. They look like other lipsticks, but contain only twenty percent of the color. They allow you to wear the shades you love, with less intensity. For a more transparent look, simply use gloss alone.

PROTIP If you are one of the many women with uneven lip color, dab foundation on your lips, blot, and apply lipstick as usual.

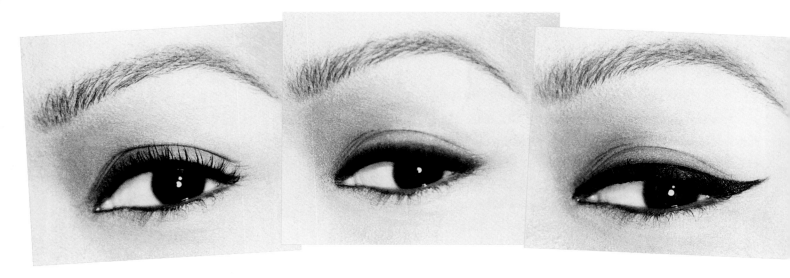

With so many forms of eyeliner available, how do I know which one to choose?

Choosing an eyeliner depends on the type of line you want. Pencils can give either soft or sharp lines. They're the easiest to handle, which makes them perfect for beginners. Liquids provide a more precise line, but applying them takes a sure and steady hand. There are also felt-tip liners, which offer the best of both worlds: the sharp definition of conventional liquid liner with the control of a pencil. Powder is yet another option. When teamed with an angled brush, it can create a soft, smoky line. Now that you know the differences, as well as the wonderful results you can achieve, the choice is yours.

EYELINER

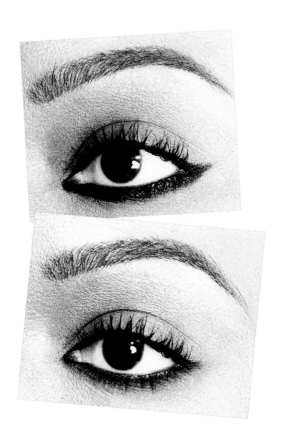

Is lining my bottom lid dated?

The whole idea behind eyeliner is to emphasize the lash line. What can make eyeliner look dated is the way in which it's applied. If you're still lining your eyes to look like Cleopatra, stop! Then start using a dark eye shadow on the bottom lids (applied with your angled brush) for a softer look. Not only is this a more subtle way to line your eyes, but you don't have to worry that the eye shadow will smudge, the way waxy pencils can.

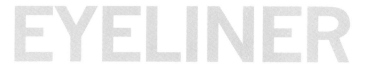

PROTIP White liner is one of the oldest—yet newest—makeup tricks in the book. Applied to the rim of the eye, it gives the appearance of wider, whiter eyes.

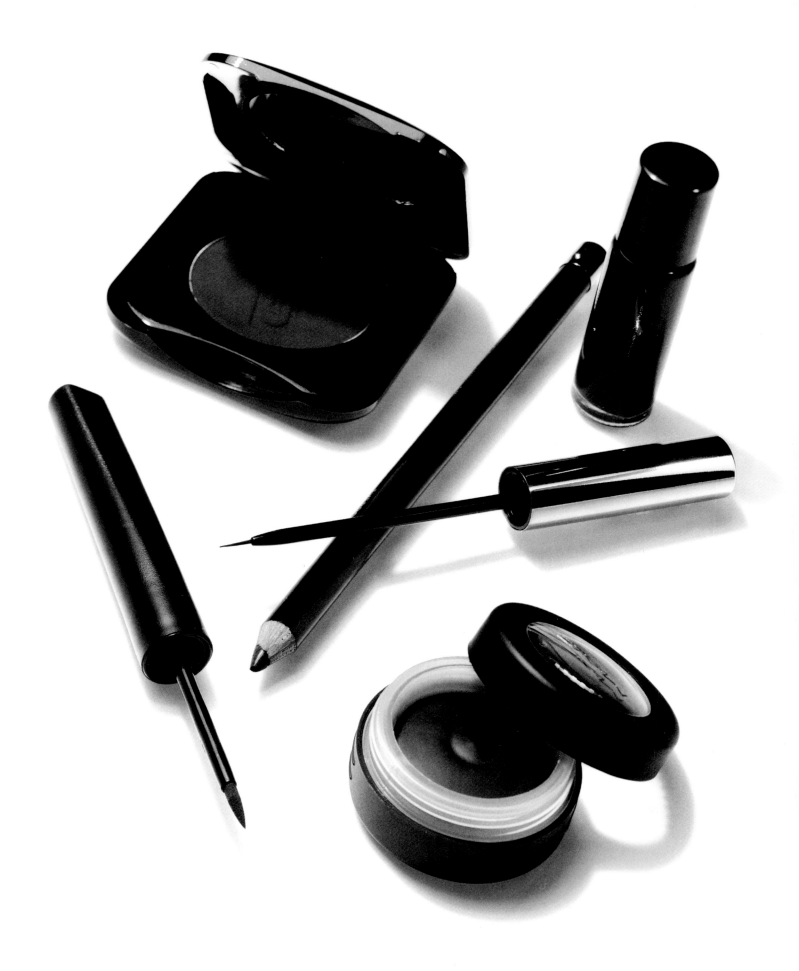

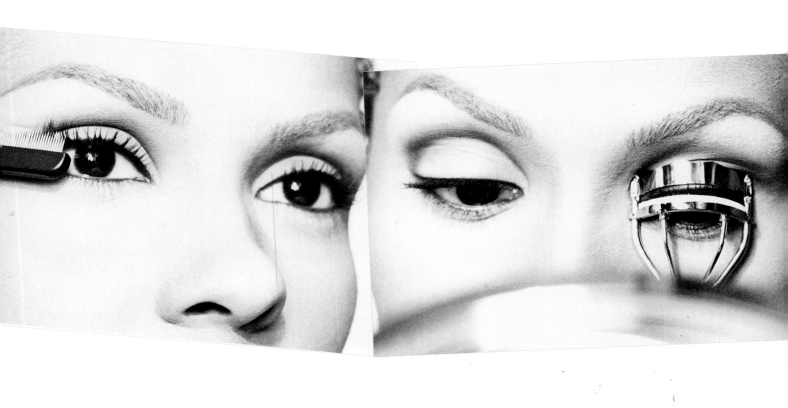

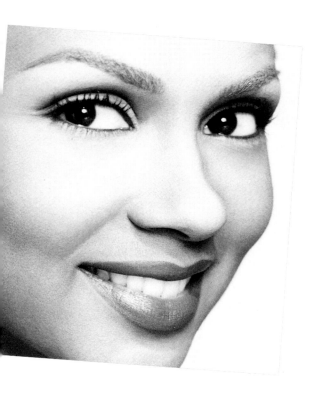

What's the best way to apply mascara?

Of all the makeup you use, mascara is the one thing you can't do without. Lashes naturally enhance the face, so even when you're not wearing any other makeup, brush on some mascara to play them up. Black mascara in particular looks gorgeous on all women, regardless of hair or eye color. It immediately brings the focus to the eyes. For the fullest, lushest lashes, first blot the applicator on dry tissue that's not too cottony, to avoid picking up tissue residue. Then, starting at the base of the lash, apply a first coat, wiggling the applicator from side to side for thickness, and pulling it outward for length. Allow the first coat of mascara to dry, and finish the rest of your face. Then reapply mascara as before. Finally, curl and comb your lashes, and you're out the door.

MASCARA

What's the purpose of curling and combing my lashes?

Curling the eyelashes makes them look naturally alluring. Like eyebrows, eyelashes don't all grow out perfectly, so curling helps bring uniformity to them while giving your eyes an instant lift. Combing eyelashes helps separate them, and removes any clumping that might occur after mascara is applied. These two little steps make for big, beautiful results.

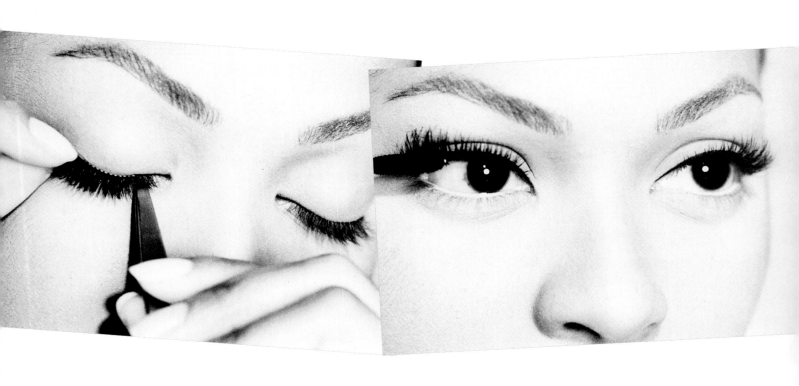

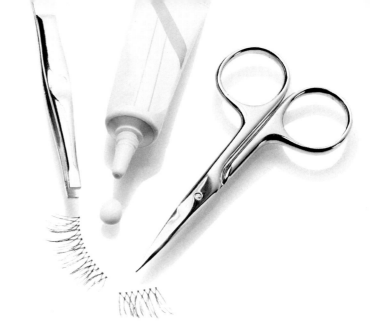

I want to try false eyelashes but don't know where to begin.

The movie starlets of Hollywood's golden era wouldn't have been caught dead without a good set of lashes, and most of the celebrities featured in this book wouldn't be without their false lashes either. Why should they be the only ones to have all the fun? For $1.99, the average cost of a set of lashes, you too can have the same glamour. Just don't wait until you're on your way to the altar, or some other big event, to master the skill of putting them on. Working with false eyelashes takes time, patience, and practice, so make sure you have plenty of all three.

Equip yourself with the necessary supplies: lashes, clear glue, cuticle scissors, and tweezers. Find natural-looking lashes that complement your own. (Steer clear of heavy lashes, unless you're performing onstage.) Measure the false lash against your own, and cut off any excess with the cuticle scissors. Next apply a thin line of glue to the band of the lash, and allow it to dry slightly, enough for it to adhere easily without sliding. Hold one end of the lash with your fingertips and the other end with your tweezers, and place it directly on top of your own lash; then push it into that very fine space where the lash grows out. Remember, the trick to making up is being able to see what goes where, so use your magnifying mirror for an even closer look.

FALSE EYELASHES

After working in the beauty biz for a number of years, I've learned that contouring and highlighting are touchy subjects for many African-American women. These techniques are often misinterpreted as refining the features to the point of denying them. If this is what you've always thought, I ask you to erase the notion from your mind and reconsider these makeup tricks for what they really are: ways to define the face. Contouring and highlighting are techniques to use when you're ready to go one step further. They're the icing on the cake. I recommend them for special occasions like weddings, proms, or evening galas, times when you're more likely to be photographed. When you've applied foundation and powder, you've taken the natural highs (the places where you naturally glow) and lows (the areas where you are naturally darker) away from your complexion. Contouring and highlighting bring those shadows and lighter areas back to the face in a more controlled manner.

CONTOURS

Start with loose powder one shade lighter than the one used to set your foundation. Apply it with a wedge sponge to the T zone, the area that's always lighter; this is a guide for contouring other parts of your face as well. With your contour brush, sweep deeper shades of pressed powder under your cheekbones, down the sides of your nose, and near your hairline, for soft yet subtle shading. If you feel you've gone too far, and you look like a character in *Cats,* dust loose powder over any of these areas to soften the effect.

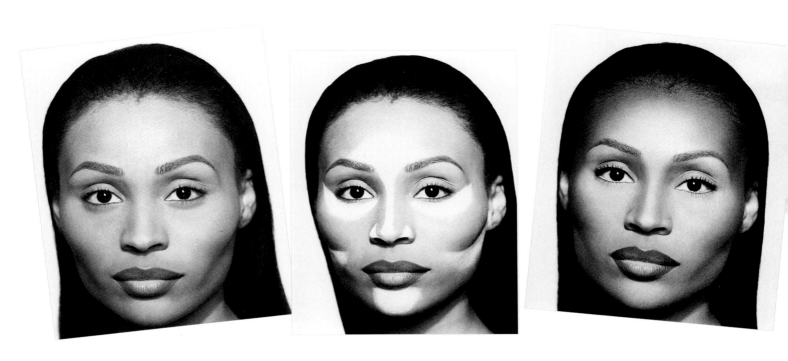

AND HIGHLIGHTS

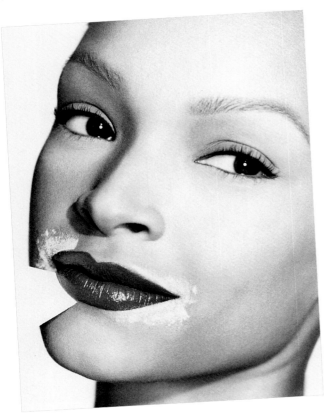

How can I keep my lipstick from bleeding?

Lipstick bleeding outside the lines is not a pretty sight, but it's nothing a little powder can't fix. With wedge sponge in hand, apply powder to the corners of your mouth, where bleeding usually occurs. This might remind you of eating a powdered doughnut, but what a difference it makes. Whisk away powder with the clean end of your sponge, and your lipstick will no longer overstep its boundaries.

How can I make my lipstick last longer?

Wouldn't it be great if you could go the entire day eating, drinking, and even kissing with your lipstick intact? Well, you can. First liberally apply your favorite shade of lipstick. Then place a tissue over your mouth, blotting all the while. Dust loose powder on top of the tissue with a powder brush, in order to set the lipstick. Remove the tissue, then reapply lipstick. There you have it—beautiful color with staying power.

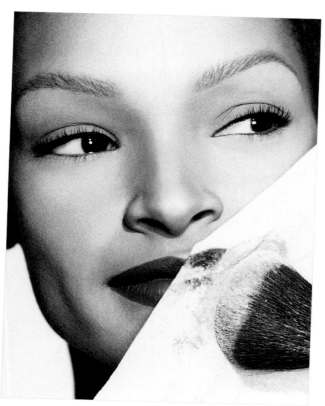

I like the color of my lip liner. Is it okay to use it as a lipstick?

Sure it is. Just don't forget to spread a little lip balm on first to avoid dragging a dry lip pencil across your mouth. Then blot. This technique can leave you with a subtle matte finish, or you can take it one step further by layering your favorite lip gloss over it.

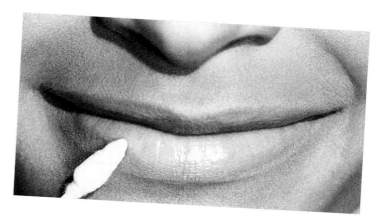

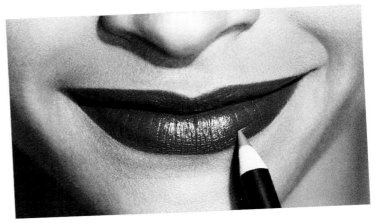

LIP TRICKS

SAVING FACE

You can't create great art without a clean canvas. It's not enough to know how to apply makeup like a pro; you must also know how to remove it like one. And you *absolutely* must remove it before going to bed. (Late nights are no excuse.) You should already be accustomed to cleaning, toning, and moisturizing, but don't rely on your cleanser alone to take makeup off completely. Whether you wear very little makeup or go all-out, your cleansing system should include a makeup remover. Start by finding a formula that suits your needs. Makeup must first be dissolved, so that it lifts off your skin easily. Leave the remover on your face while you brush your teeth or draw your bath. The skin around the eyes is extremely delicate, so it's important here to use a remover specifically for this area. Above all, remember to be gentle. If you tug and pull at your skin, you are asking for trouble later. Taking good care of your skin goes beyond any beauty benefits that makeup can deliver. Be good to your skin, and it will be good to you.

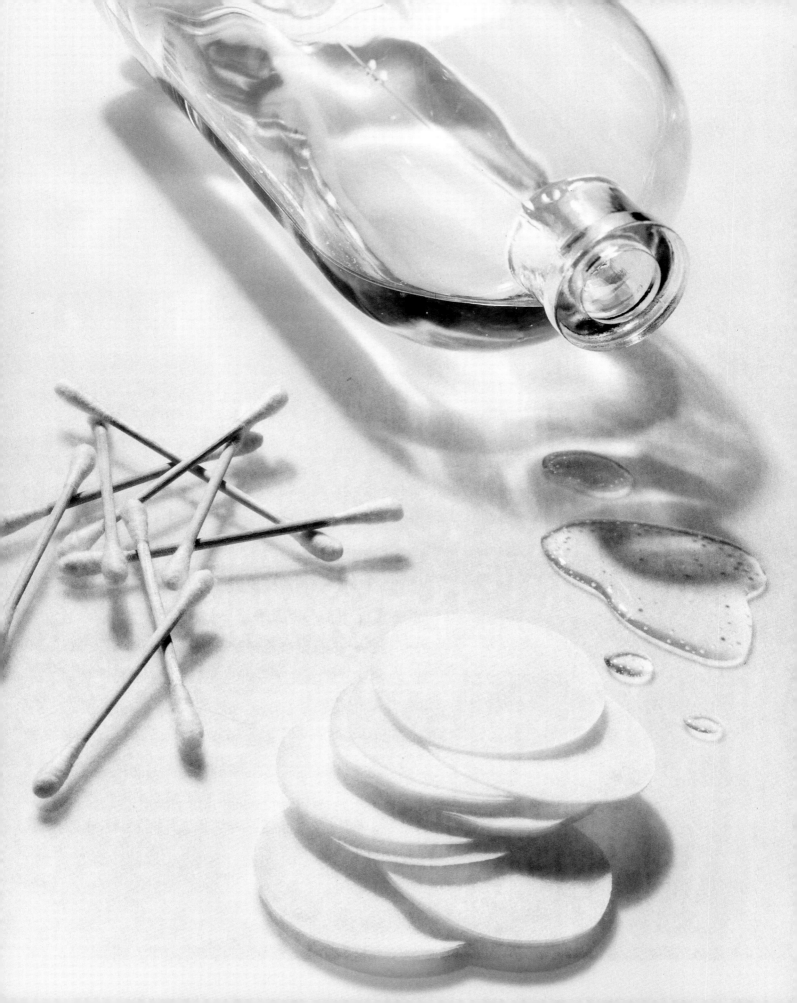

"PEOPLE WERE CALLING MY SURGEON WAS DR. FINE— I GUARANTEE HE'LL YEARS OFF YOUR

AND ASKING ME WHO
WAS. I SAID IT
SAM FINE, THAT IS!
TAKE AT LEAST TEN
FACE, LIKE HE DID MINE!"

PATTI LaBELLE

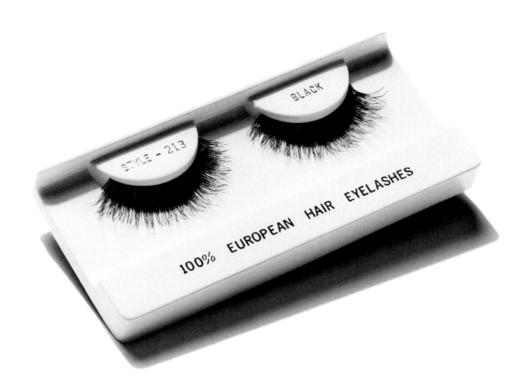

MAKEOVERS

HAVE YOU EVER

STOPPED TO WONDER

how you'd look if you wore a different shade of lipstick, lightened your eyebrows, or used eye shadow in a dramatic new way? Consider a makeover. It's a wonderful opportunity to explore the many options makeup has to offer. But don't let the word "makeover" scare you. It's not as permanent as it may sound; it's simply a different approach to makeup from the one you're accustomed to. And if you haven't experienced the wonders of makeup, it's an excellent introduction. Best of all, if you aren't happy with the results, you can always wash it off and start over. For a total transformation, look to professional makeup artists. With their trained eye and expertise, they can help you gain a new perspective. Take advantage of the makeup artists' services offered by many cosmetics lines. (Remember, that's where I got my start.) Or become your own makeup artist, by sampling new products and colors to further your cosmetics know-how.

The women on the following pages represent different beauty styles, and different needs and desires. With looks ranging from clean and natural to full-fledged glamour, these models exemplify the possibilities out there waiting for you.

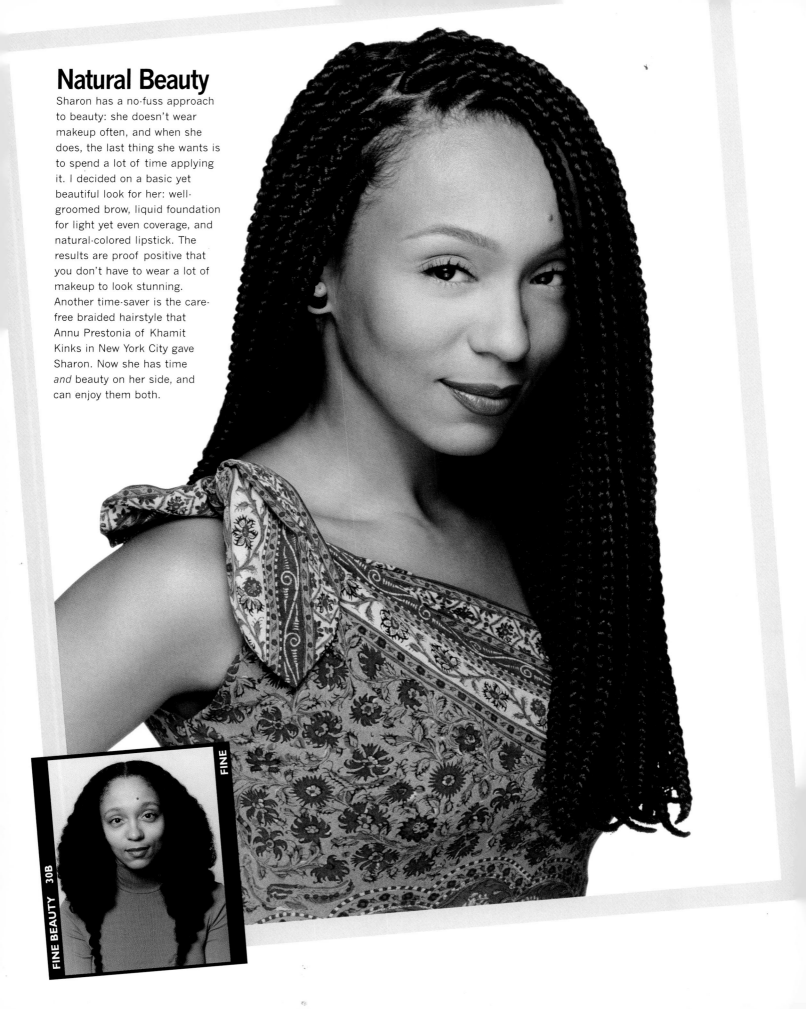

Natural Beauty

Sharon has a no-fuss approach to beauty: she doesn't wear makeup often, and when she does, the last thing she wants is to spend a lot of time applying it. I decided on a basic yet beautiful look for her: well-groomed brow, liquid foundation for light yet even coverage, and natural-colored lipstick. The results are proof positive that you don't have to wear a lot of makeup to look stunning. Another time-saver is the care-free braided hairstyle that Annu Prestonia of Khamit Kinks in New York City gave Sharon. Now she has time *and* beauty on her side, and can enjoy them both.

FINE

FINE BEAUTY 30B

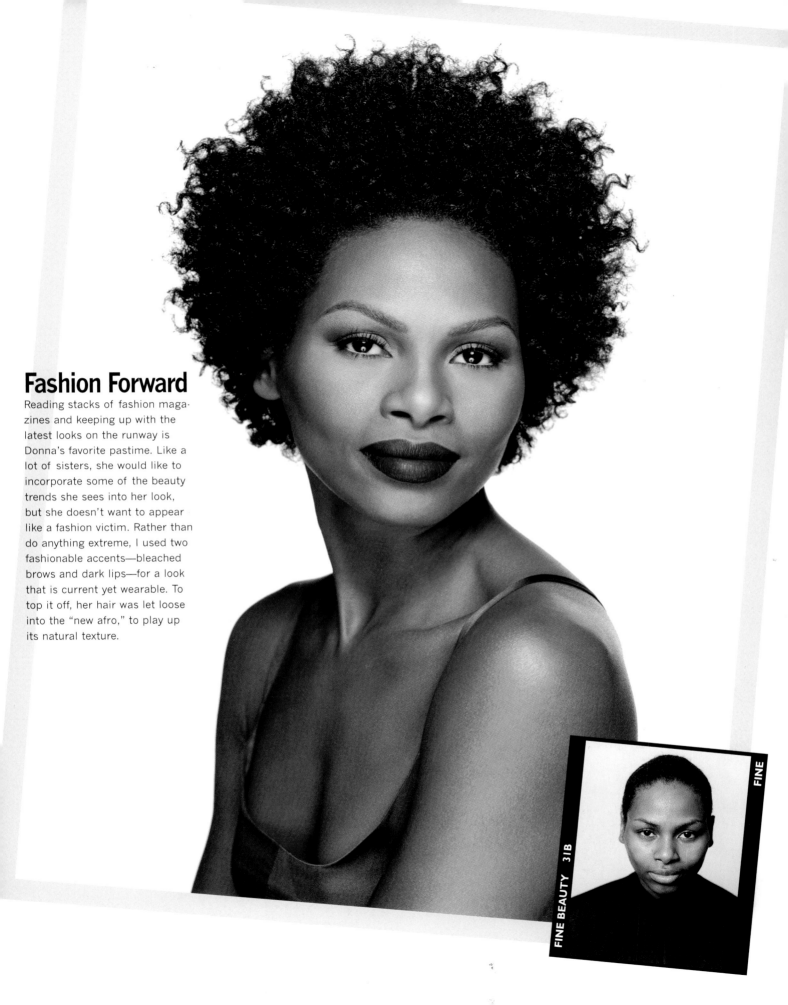

Fashion Forward

Reading stacks of fashion magazines and keeping up with the latest looks on the runway is Donna's favorite pastime. Like a lot of sisters, she would like to incorporate some of the beauty trends she sees into her look, but she doesn't want to appear like a fashion victim. Rather than do anything extreme, I used two fashionable accents—bleached brows and dark lips—for a look that is current yet wearable. To top it off, her hair was let loose into the "new afro," to play up its natural texture.

FINE BEAUTY 318

FINE

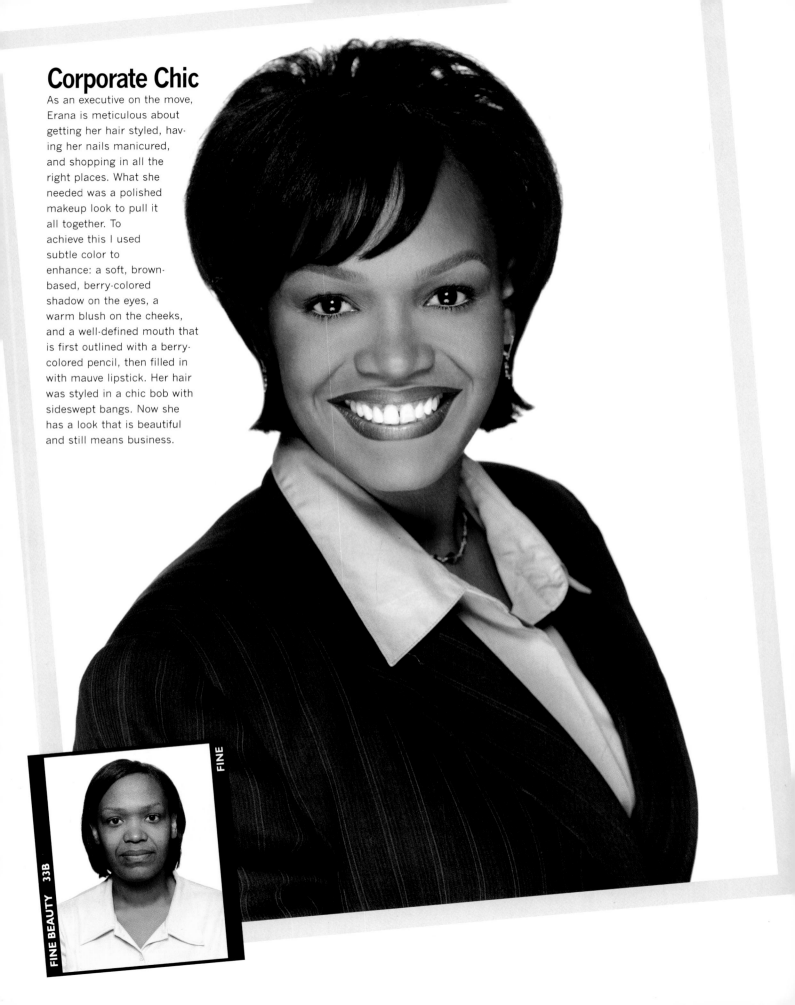

Corporate Chic

As an executive on the move, Erana is meticulous about getting her hair styled, having her nails manicured, and shopping in all the right places. What she needed was a polished makeup look to pull it all together. To achieve this I used subtle color to enhance: a soft, brown-based, berry-colored shadow on the eyes, a warm blush on the cheeks, and a well-defined mouth that is first outlined with a berry-colored pencil, then filled in with mauve lipstick. Her hair was styled in a chic bob with sideswept bangs. Now she has a look that is beautiful and still means business.

FINE

FINE BEAUTY   33B

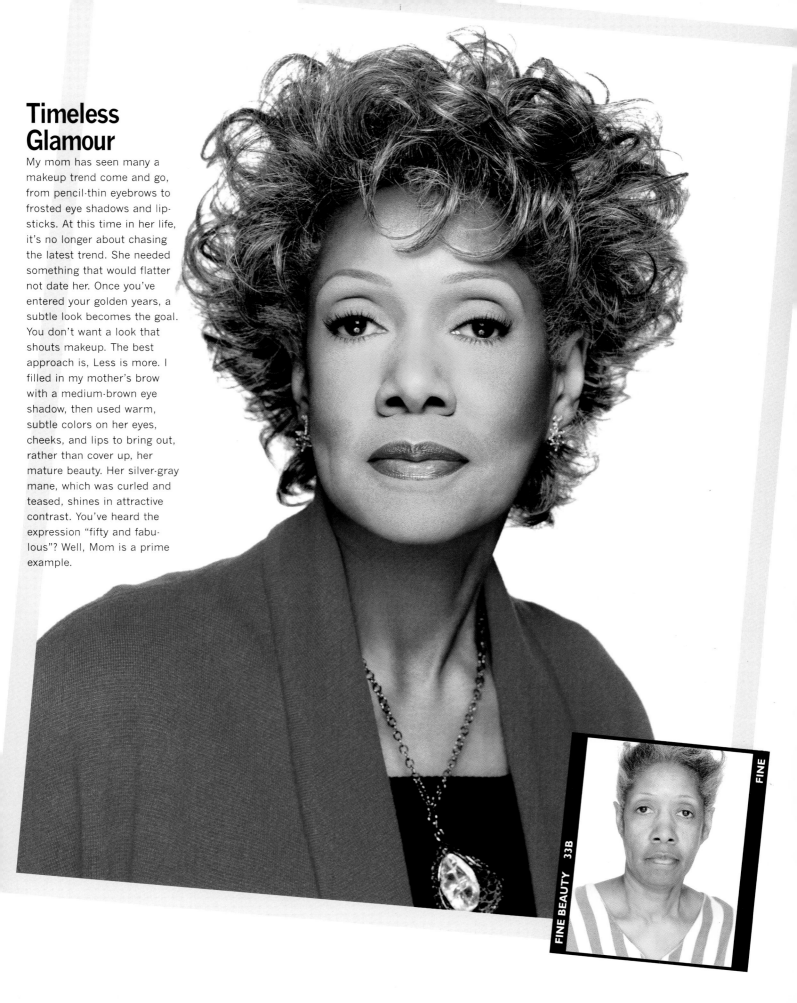

Timeless Glamour

My mom has seen many a makeup trend come and go, from pencil-thin eyebrows to frosted eye shadows and lipsticks. At this time in her life, it's no longer about chasing the latest trend. She needed something that would flatter not date her. Once you've entered your golden years, a subtle look becomes the goal. You don't want a look that shouts makeup. The best approach is, Less is more. I filled in my mother's brow with a medium-brown eye shadow, then used warm, subtle colors on her eyes, cheeks, and lips to bring out, rather than cover up, her mature beauty. Her silver-gray mane, which was curled and teased, shines in attractive contrast. You've heard the expression "fifty and fabulous"? Well, Mom is a prime example.

FINE BEAUTY 33B

FINE

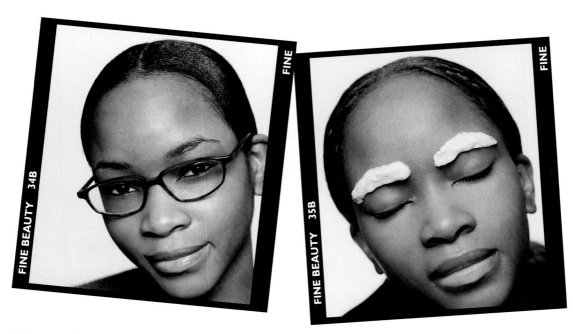

Model Changes

Marie is in a business of constant change. As a model, she can be seen strutting down a catwalk sporting blond hair one day, dark brown the next. She knows the glowing results that change can bring, so I went for a look packed with knockout appeal. First I bleached her eyebrows to match the golden streaks of color applied to her hair. Then I traded her glasses for colored contact lenses to set off her already dazzling eyes. I capped it with my favorite beauty accessory: false eyelashes. Without a doubt, Marie is ready for her close-up.

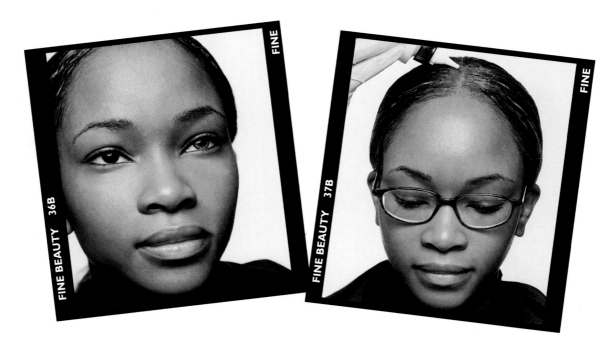

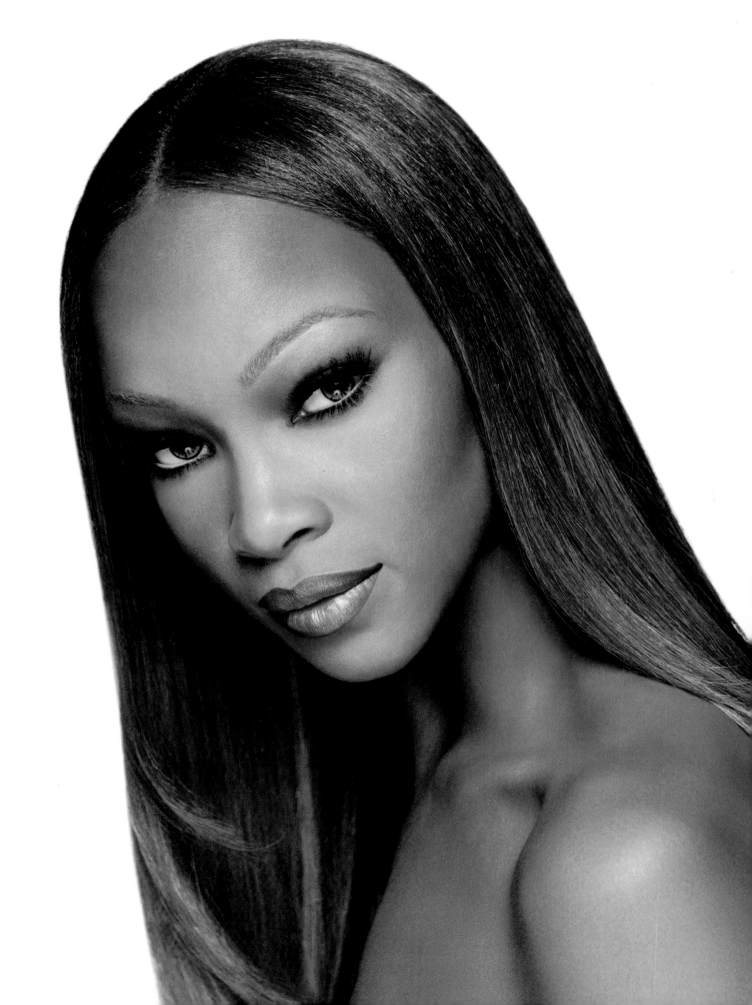

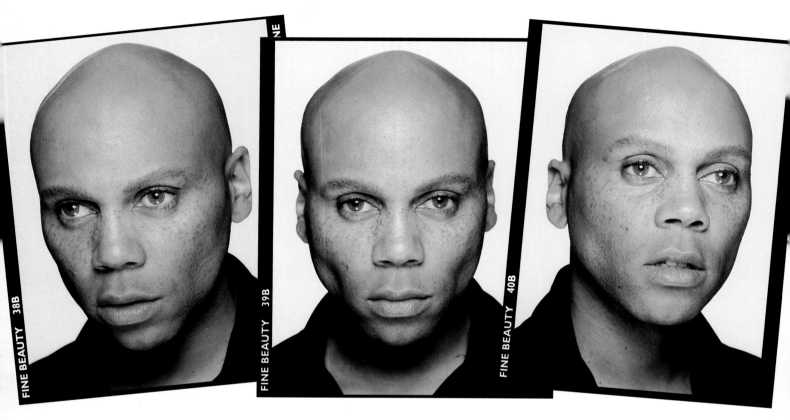

FINE BEAUTY 38B

FINE BEAUTY 39B

FINE BEAUTY 40B

Maximum Glamour

If making up is fun, then RuPaul is having a blast. The man gives nothing but good face. For him, putting on false eyelashes is second nature. He can line his lips with his eyes closed and pull on his drag in record time. No wonder he's "Supermodel of the World." Working on RuPaul is a makeup artist's dream: there is little he won't do to maximize his glamour potential. I invited this "transformer extraordinaire" to be one of my makeovers not just because his transformation is the most radical, but because his approach to making up is a perfect demonstration of the wonderful possibilities makeup offers. So the next time you're preparing for a night out on the town, remember RuPaul's sound advice: "You better work!"

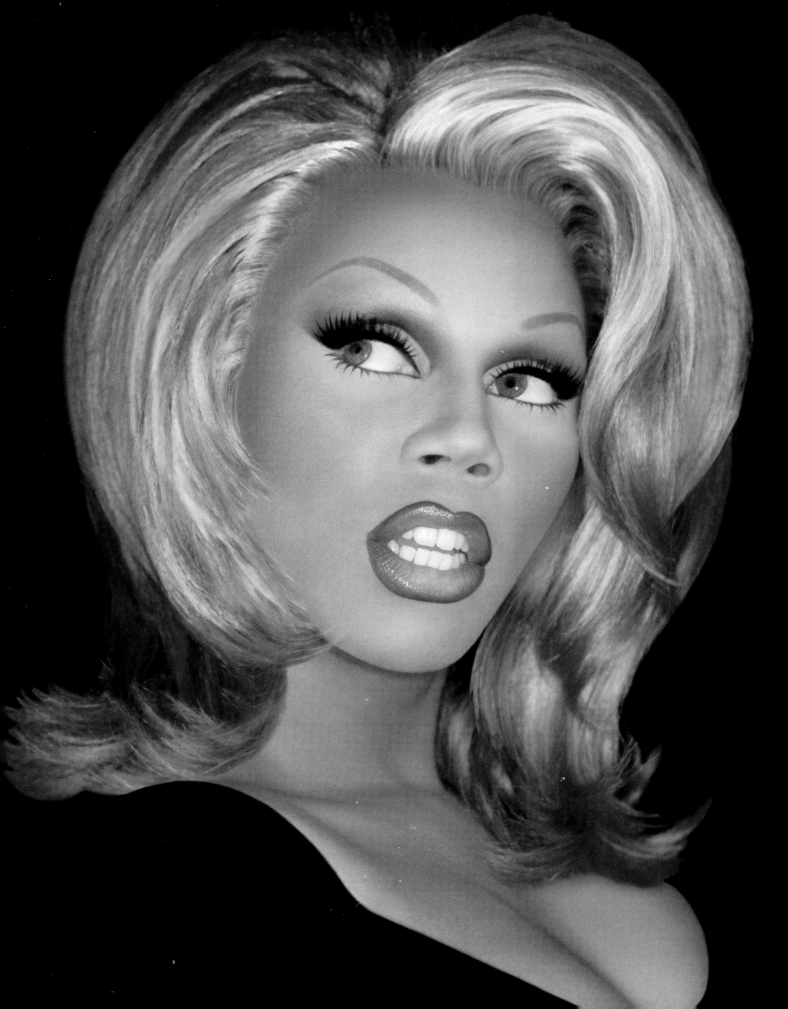

"I LOVE FOR SAM TO
WHEN HE DOES MY
BEAUTIFUL. I CAN'T

MAKE ME UP FOR VIDEOS.
FACE HE MAKES ME FEEL
STAY OUT OF THE MIRROR."

BRANDY

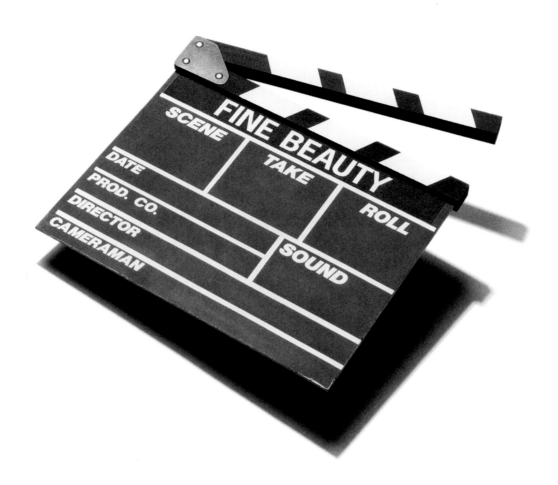

FINE BEAUTY

SCENE   TAKE

DATE

PROD. CO.   ROLL

DIRECTOR

CAMERAMAN   SOUND

VIDEO SOUL

NOWADAYS, INSTEAD

OF FLIPPING THE PAGES OF

magazines, many people look to music videos and commercials in search of the latest trends in fashion, hair, and makeup. I've had the extreme pleasure of applying my skills on several of these mini-musicals. The days can be long, and the pressure is on to get things right on the first take. However, videos offer yet another exciting way for me to express my artistic talent, while I contribute to music history. Along with the standard tools of the trade, I always carry my camera to document the fun and good times. Here I've included some celebrity snapshots and images from my favorite videos to give you a peek at what you don't see on screen. Enjoy!

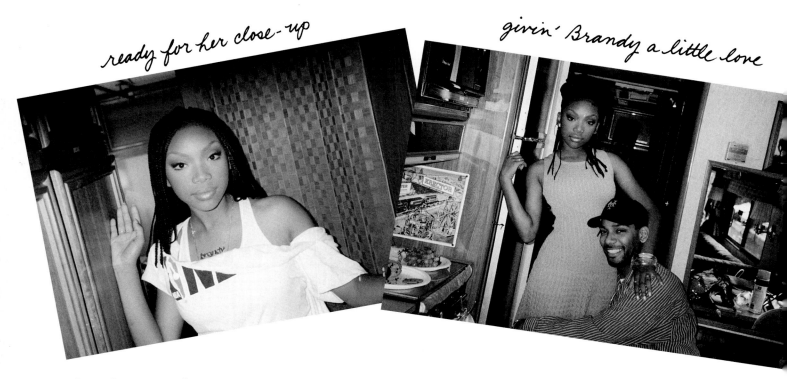

ready for her close-up

givin' Brandy a little love

Brokenhearted

The beautiful remixed version of this song, featuring Wanya Morris of the hit group Boyz II Men, catapulted Brandy to another level. Where she had come across as a lovestruck teenager in her earlier releases, by the time of this single she had blossomed into a young woman singing about the heartaches of love. For the video she introduced an alluring new look, complete with glamorous makeup and designer clothes. Who knew being brokenhearted could look this good?

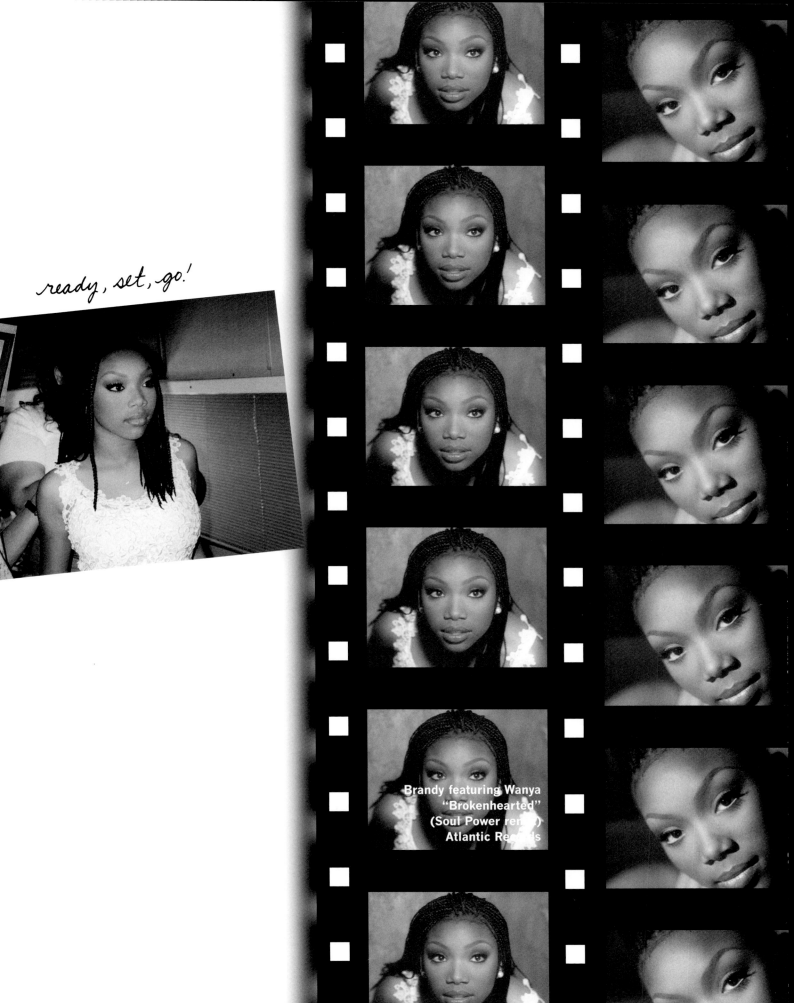

ready, set, go!

Brandy featuring Wanya
"Brokenhearted"
(Soul Power remix)
Atlantic Records

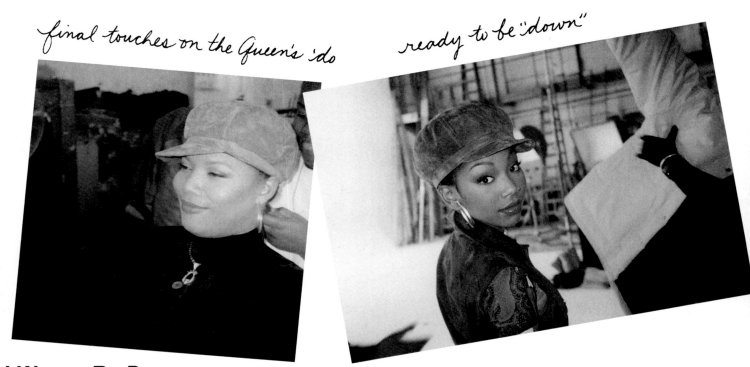

final touches on the Queen's 'do

ready to be "down"

I Wanna Be Down

As if Brandy's single "I Wanna Be Down" hadn't been a big enough hit when it debuted, after it was remixed it went through the roof. That's because some of the biggest female names in hip-hop added their unique flavor to this effort. Accompanying the youthful, fresh-faced Brandy was the streetwise MC Lyte, the sexy-with-an-edge Yo Yo, and the self-assured Queen Latifah. My challenge for the video was to bring out their beauty without compromising their individual styles. But each of them came to my chair with an open mind and a willingness to let me work my magic, so I was able to pull it off effortlessly.

me and my Yo Yo

Brandy featuring MC
Queen Latifah, and
"I Wanna Be Down" (re
Atlantic Records

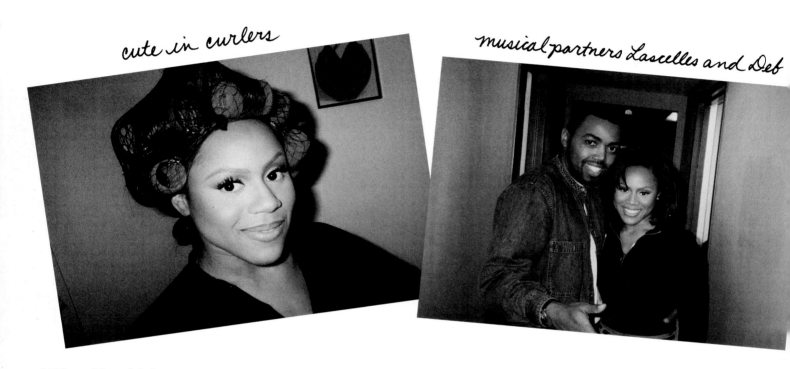

cute in curlers

musical partners Lascelles and Deb

Who Do U Love

I had the pleasure of working with Deborah Cox on the video for her first single, "Sentimental," as well as the video for her second release, "Who Do U Love." After Arista Records' president, Clive Davis (the force behind Whitney Houston and Aretha Franklin), heard this Canadian beauty, he immediately signed her to his roster. It's always exciting to work with up-and-coming artists. They bring fresh and exuberant energy to their endeavors, and Deborah's no exception. And she has a great voice, and a personality to match. I'd work with her any day.

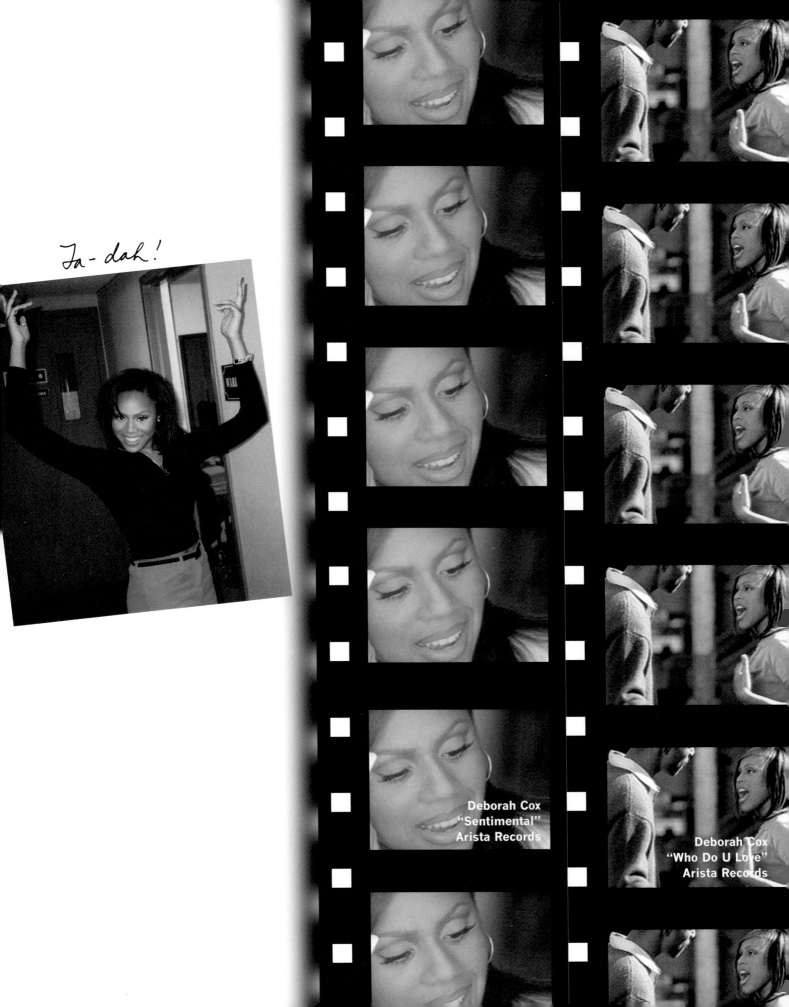

Ta-dah!

Deborah Cox
"Sentimental"
Arista Records

Deborah Cox
"Who Do U Love"
Arista Records

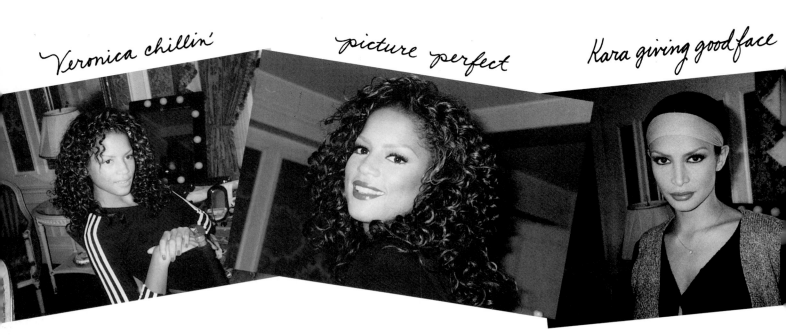

Veronica chillin' *picture perfect* *Kara giving good face*

Freek'n You

Director Brett Ratner served up high fashion for this sexy video. Shot on location in a luxe penthouse and featuring top models Veronica Webb, Beverly Peele, Kara Young, and Lana Ogilvy, it was an opportunity for a reunion with my runway buddies. Models are natural performers, but these four worked it like the song was their own, emoting to the hilt. This was one fierce video!

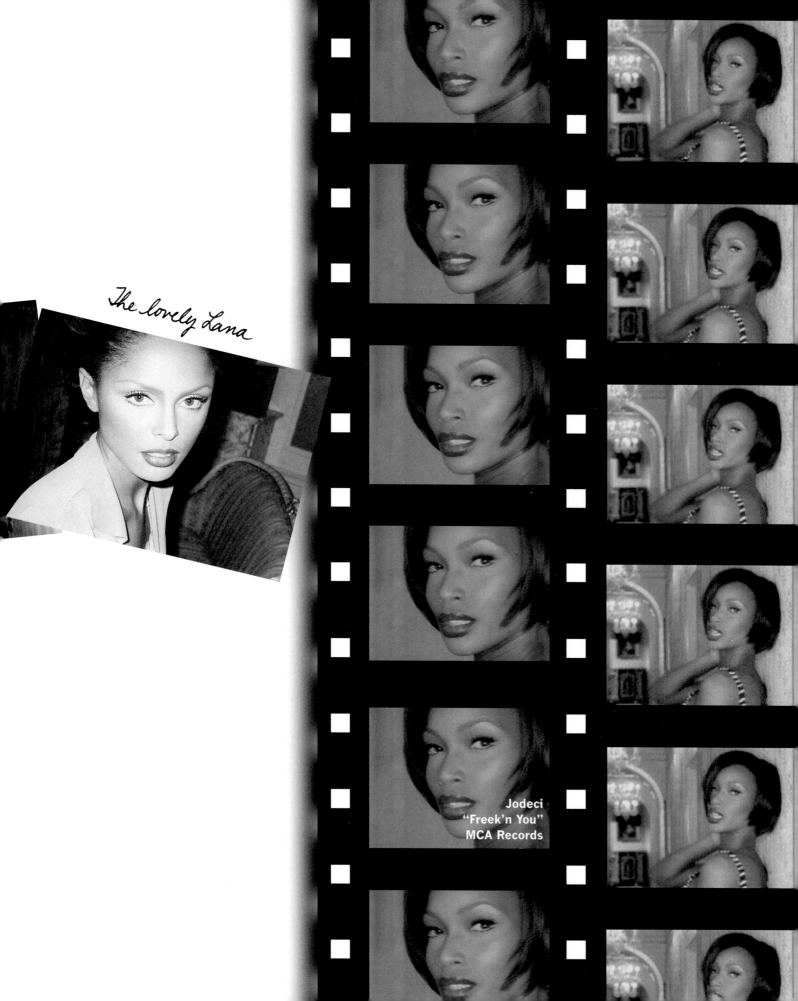

The lovely Lana

Jodeci
"Freek'n You"
MCA Records

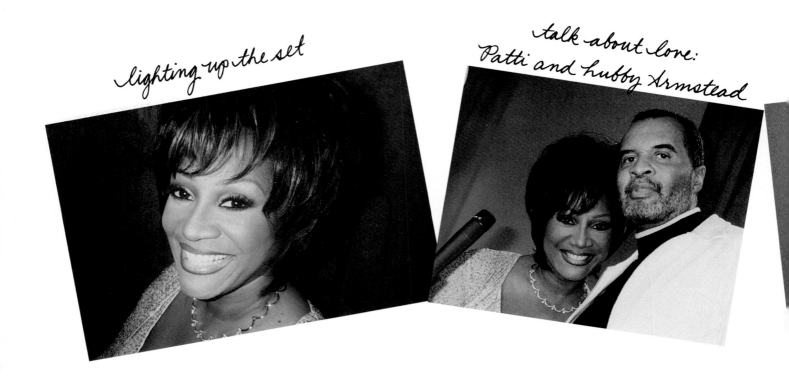

lighting up the set

talk about love: Patti and hubby Armstead

When You Talk About Love

Whenever Patti LaBelle performs, it's a virtual "love fest." Whether she's fixing her sweet mouth to "Talk About Love," or looking for the "Right Kinda Lover," she lets the good times roll, and it's a ball for everyone involved. Have you noticed how she seems to get younger-looking with each new video? That's all that spirited energy acting in her favor. The prerequisite for working with her? Say her name: "Patti, Patti!"

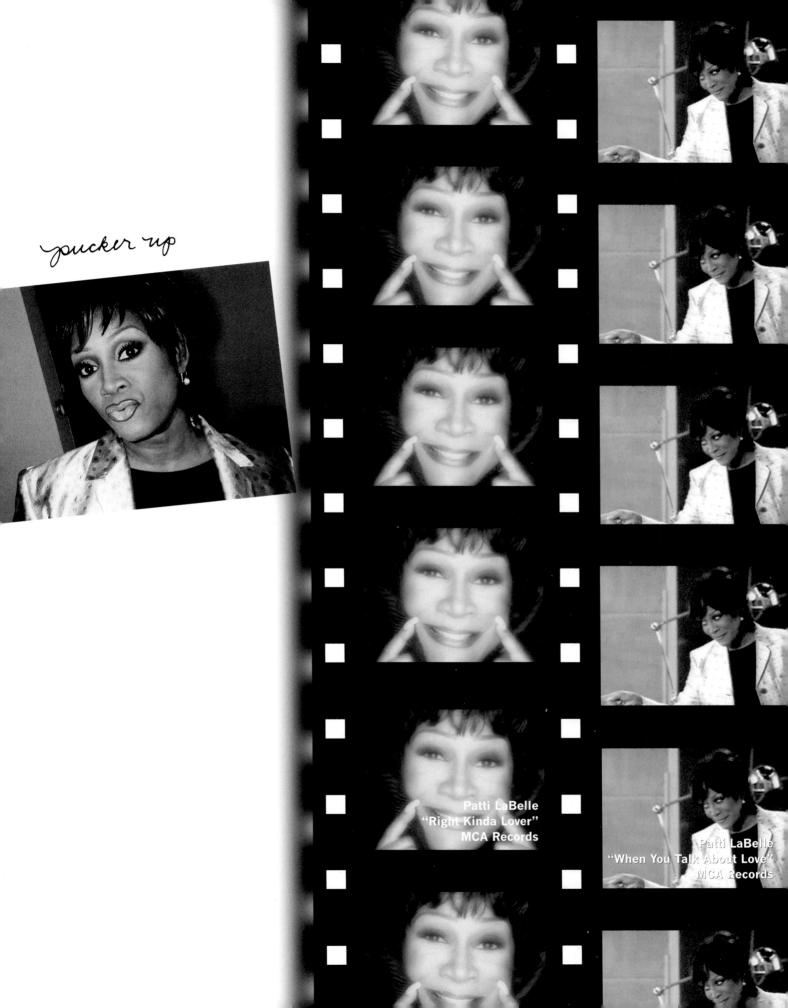

pucker up

Patti LaBelle
"Right Kinda Lover"
MCA Records

Patti LaBelle
"When You Talk About Love"
MCA Records

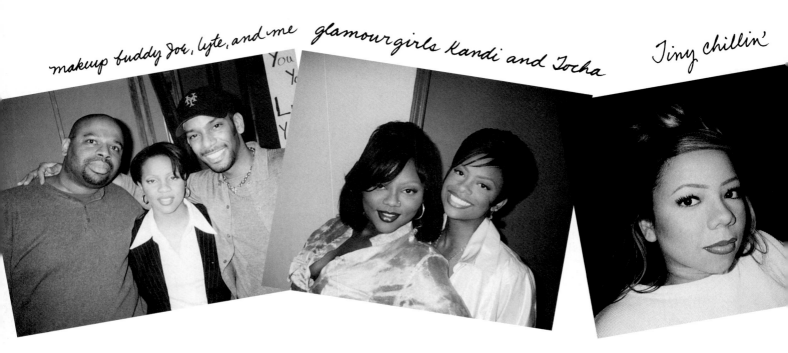

makeup buddy Joe, Lyte, and me   glamourgirls Kandi and Tocha   Tiny chillin'

Keep On, Keepin' On

Videos are usually pretty grueling all-day affairs. But in "Keep On, Keepin' On," the party atmosphere you see on screen is a reflection of the good time we had on the set. All of these ladies were such a pleasure to work with that the video hardly felt like a job. MC Lyte sported a glamorous new look that included tailored suits and a stylish bob haircut (I don't think she's looking for a roughneck anymore). And best of all, this won a Soul Train Music Award for Best Video. It's always nice to see your efforts pay off.

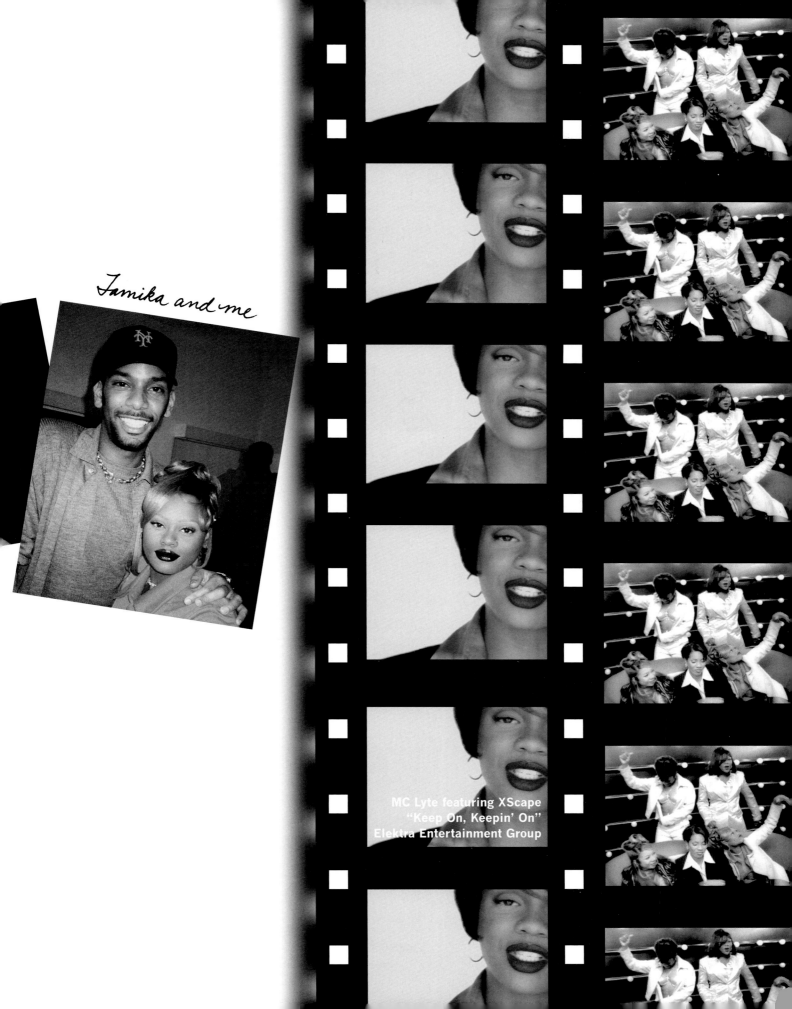

Tamika and me

MC Lyte featuring XScape
"Keep On, Keepin' On"
Elektra Entertainment Group

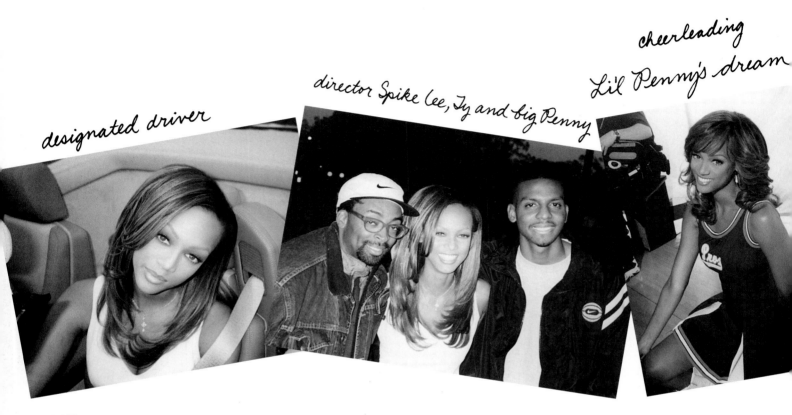

designated driver

director Spike Lee, Ty and big Penny

cheerleading Li'l Penny's dream

Nike

Tyra might be the only supermodel in the world with a wooden puppet as an avid admirer. As you probably know from the popular Nike ad campaign, Li'l Penny has been pursuing her since he first spotted her. He was so taken with Tyra that she became the subject of his basketball dreams, cheering him on and blowing him kisses on the court. What could possibly happen next? (Turn the page to find out.)

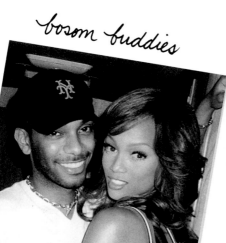

bosom buddies

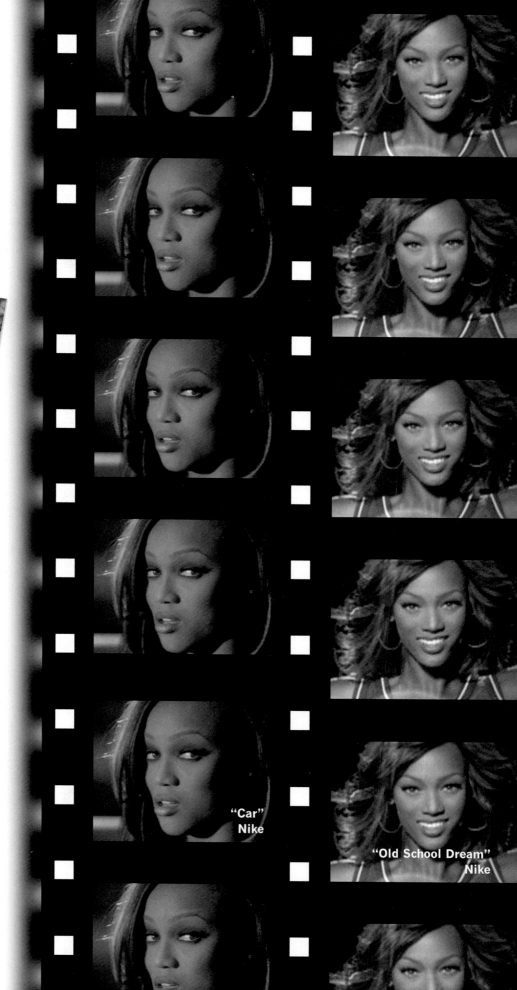

"Car"
Nike

"Old School Dream"
Nike

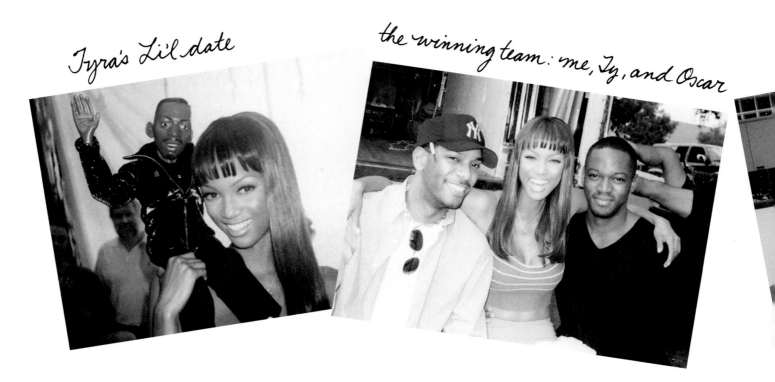

Tyra's Li'l date

the winning team: me, Ty, and Oscar

Nike

When Li'l Penny threw his Super Bowl party, everyone was in the house, from Olympic track star Michael Johnson to director Spike Lee. It was here that Li'l Penny asked for Tyra's hand in marriage. All she could muster was a look of bedazzlement. Will she be the future Mrs. Li'l Penny? Who knows? Tyra and I have worked on a lot of assignments together, but these were, hands down, the most hilarious.

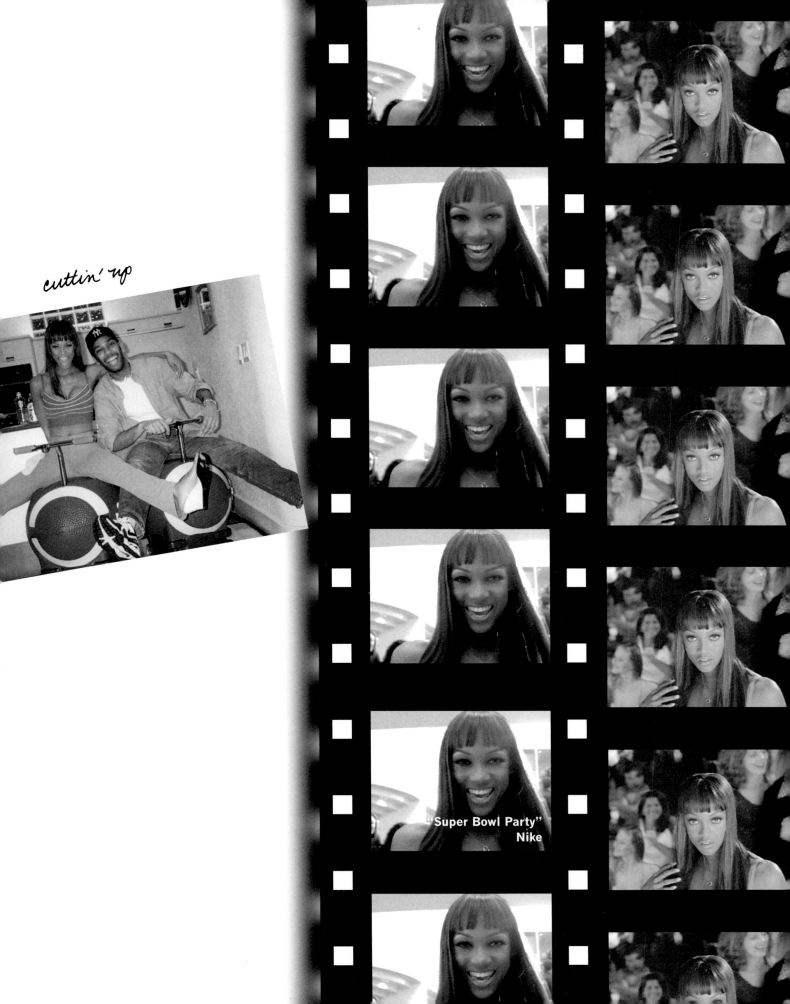

cuttin' up

"Super Bowl Party"
Nike

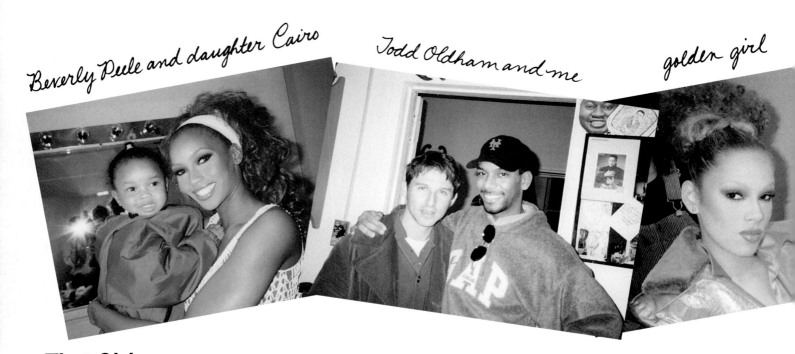

Beverly Peele and daughter Cairo

Todd Oldham and me

golden girl

That Girl

Fashion meets dance-hall reggae is the best way to describe this video. Co-directed by the talented Hype Williams and top designer Todd Oldham, it featured fabulous models strutting down a supermarket aisle that served as a catwalk, tossing groceries into their shopping carts with total abandon, as reggae artists Maxi Priest and Shaggy sang about being mesmerized by them. I can't say that I'd ever been to a grocery store like that.

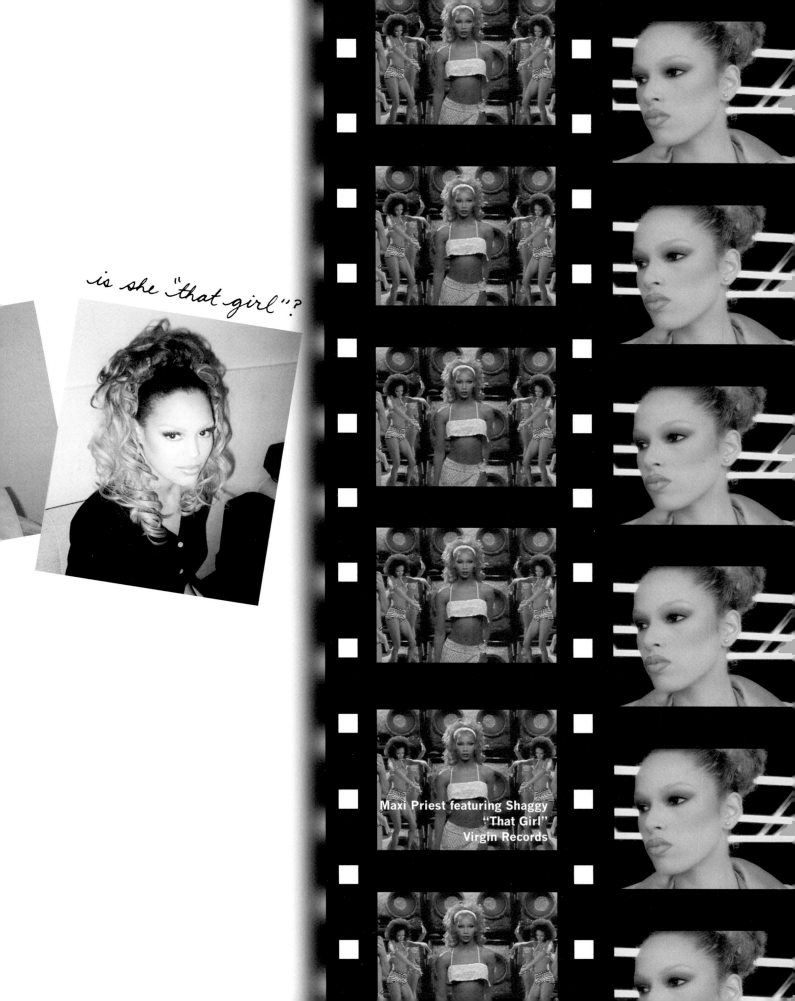

is she "that girl"?

Maxi Priest featuring Shaggy
"That Girl"
Virgin Records

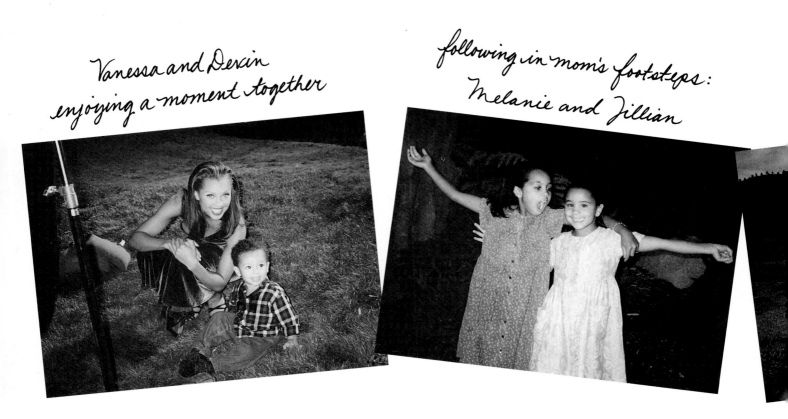

Vanessa and Devin enjoying a moment together

following in mom's footsteps: Melanie and Jillian

Colors of the Wind

It's hard to believe that the "Colors of the Wind" video, featuring Vanessa strolling through a lush forest, was shot on an indoor soundstage. Such are the wonders of Hollywood. Meanwhile, in the Big Apple, "The Sweetest Days" was shot in Central Park, as teeming crowds looked on. Vanessa performed with style and grace as usual. No one conjures up images of life's simple pleasures as lovingly as she does.

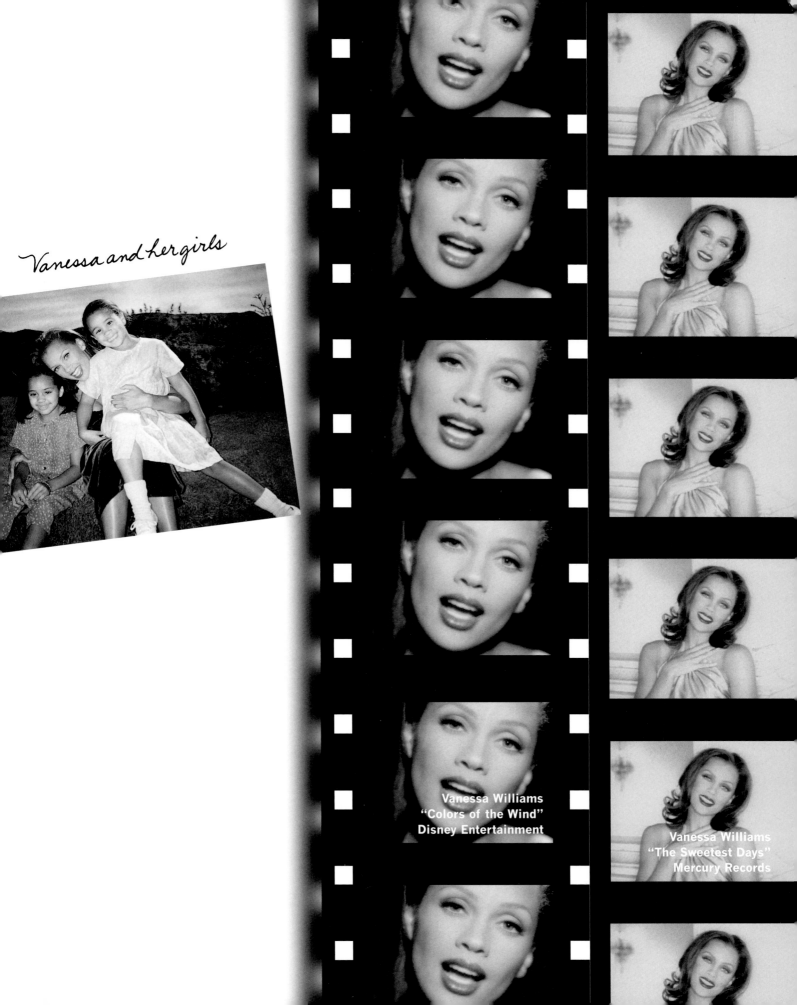

Vanessa and her girls

Vanessa Williams
"Colors of the Wind"
Disney Entertainment

Vanessa Williams
"The Sweetest Days"
Mercury Records

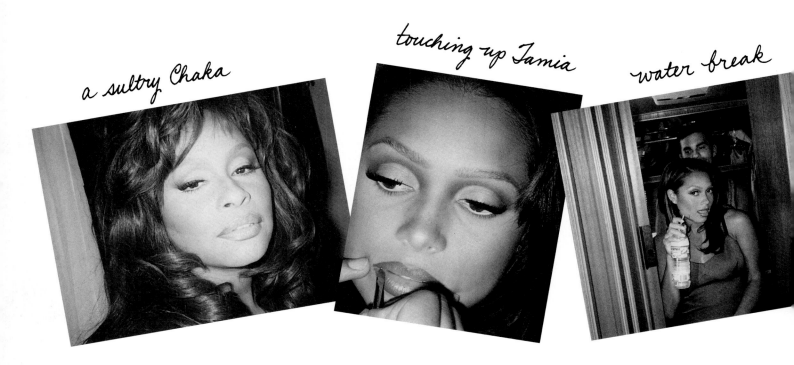

a sultry Chaka

touching up Tamia

water break

Missing You

This video required that I arrive on set to start makeup at *three a.m.* Why? So that director F. Gary Gray (who also directed the movie *Set It Off,* where the song is heard) could capture the morning light he'd envisioned. No one said this business was easy, but it all was worth it in the end. Not only did the video turn out wonderfully, it allowed me the opportunity to beautify two legendary vocalists, Gladys Knight and Chaka Khan, as well as newcomer Tamia, who is undoubtedly destined to join their ranks.

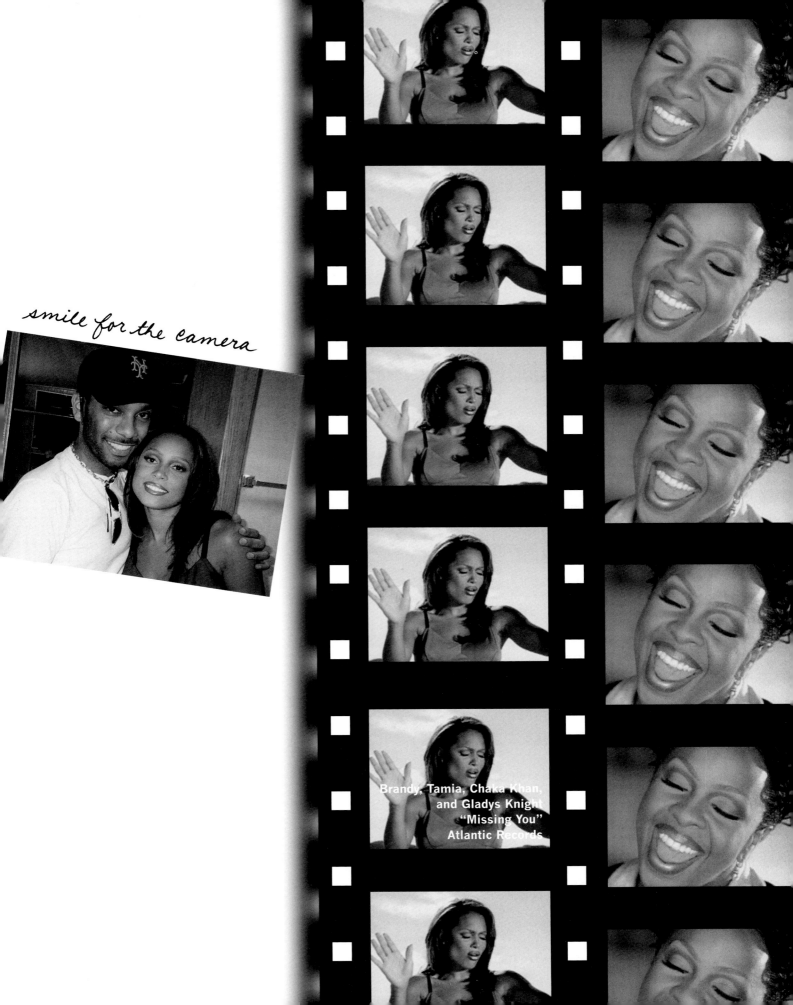

smile for the camera

Brandy, Tamia, Chaka Khan,
and Gladys Knight
"Missing You"
Atlantic Records

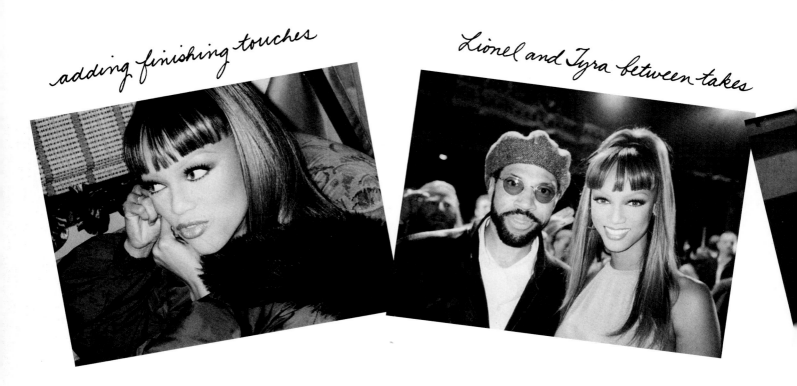

adding finishing touches

Lionel and Tyra between takes

Don't Want to Lose

When Lionel Richie needed a woman who could stir desire with just the bat of an eyelash in the video for "Don't Want to Lose," his first single in almost ten years, he chose Tyra Banks as the object of his affection. Here she plays a star on the rise, exiting limousines, ducking paparazzi, and being escorted by bodyguards while looking utterly ravishing from scene to scene (what a stretch!). She and her mother/manager both were dazzled by the video and agreed that Tyra looked her absolute best. Now *that's* a compliment, coming from a supermodel and a supermom.

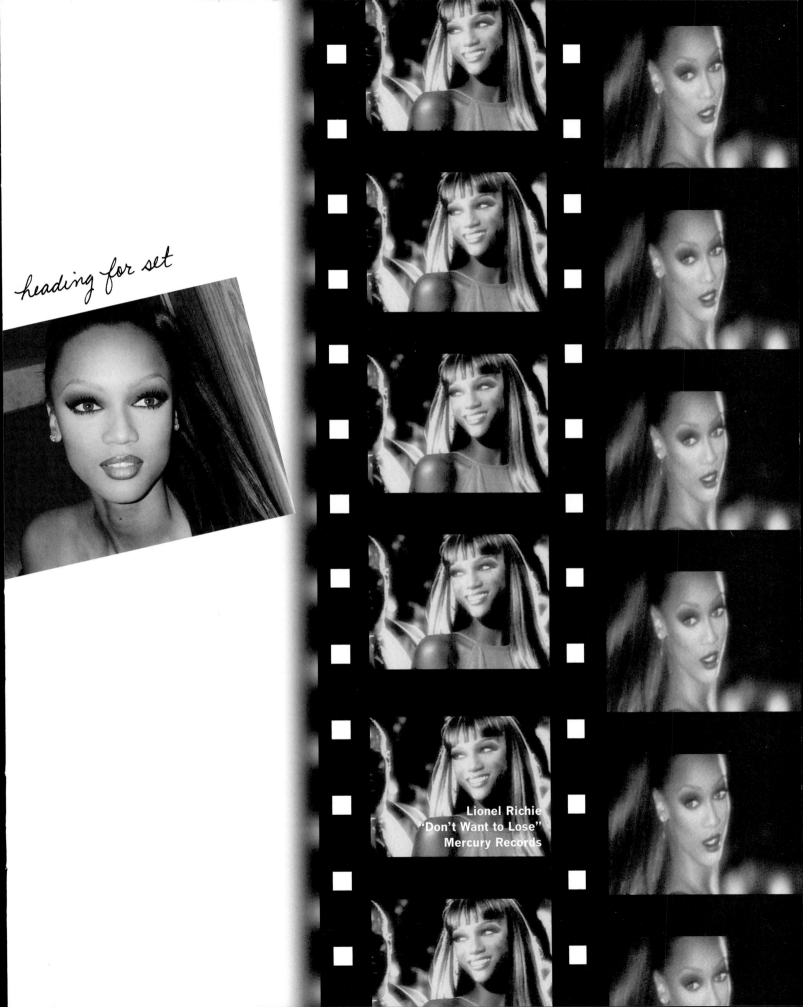

heading for set

Lionel Richie
"Don't Want to Lose"
Mercury Records

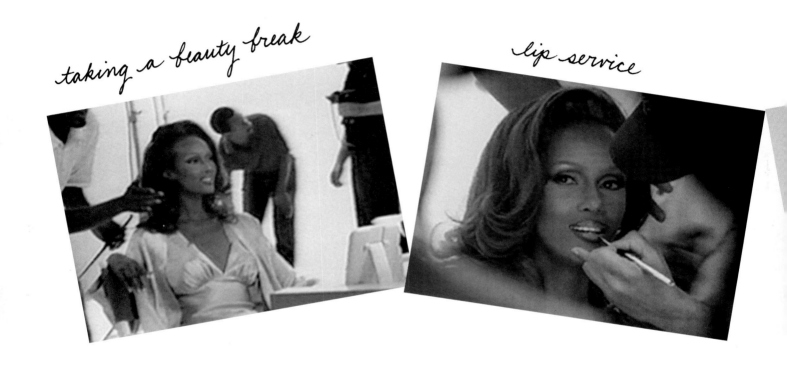

taking a beauty break

lip service

Wendy's

Fashion and fast food never exactly went hand in hand, until mega-model Iman penned a letter to her pal Dave Thomas of Wendy's to congratulate him on a chicken sandwich well done. Models have a reputation for being notorious non-eaters, but Iman shatters that myth and goes one better by delivering a sensual, mouth-watering description of this sandwich. For this ad, we spent hours doing Iman's hair and makeup, only to reenact the whole process in front of the camera. Iman had just returned to New York from a London jaunt, but jet lag was hardly a problem for this international jet-setter. As usual, she gave it her all, playing her own glamorous self.

getting it right

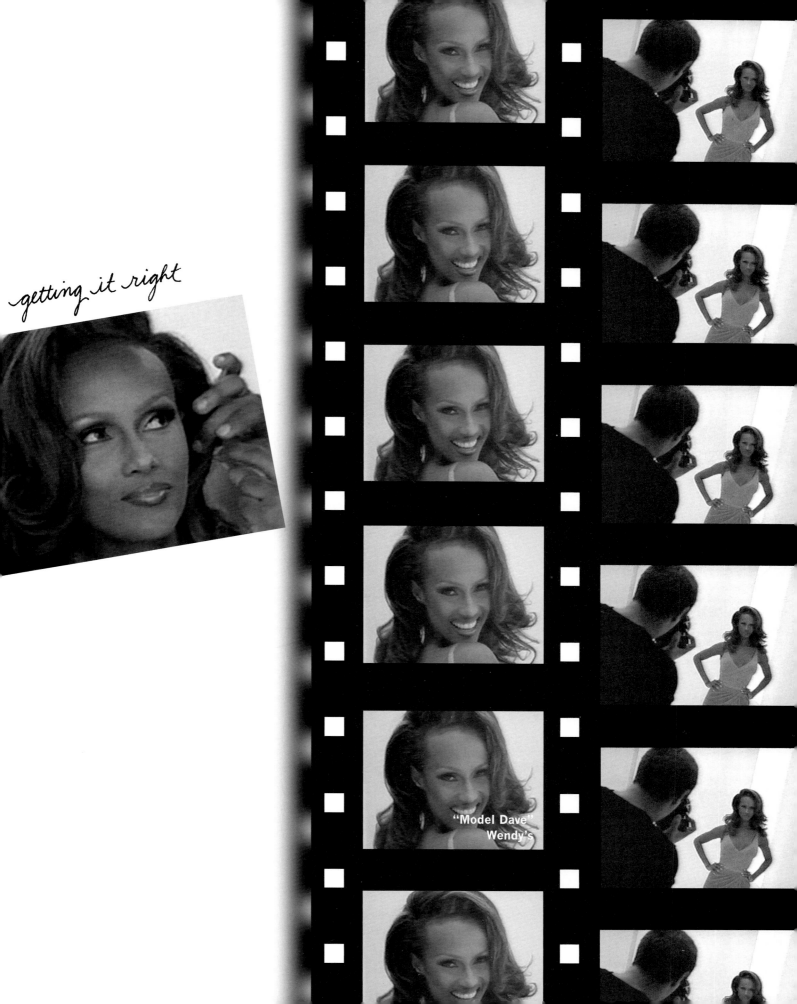

"Model Dave"
Wendy's

"SAM IS DYNAMIC, PERFECTIONIST. WITH SPONGE, YOU CAN FLAW WILL BE EVERY ASSET

A VISIONARY AND A
HIM BEHIND THE MAKEUP
TRUST THAT EVERY
HIDDEN, AND
ACCENTUATED."

VANESSA WILLIAMS

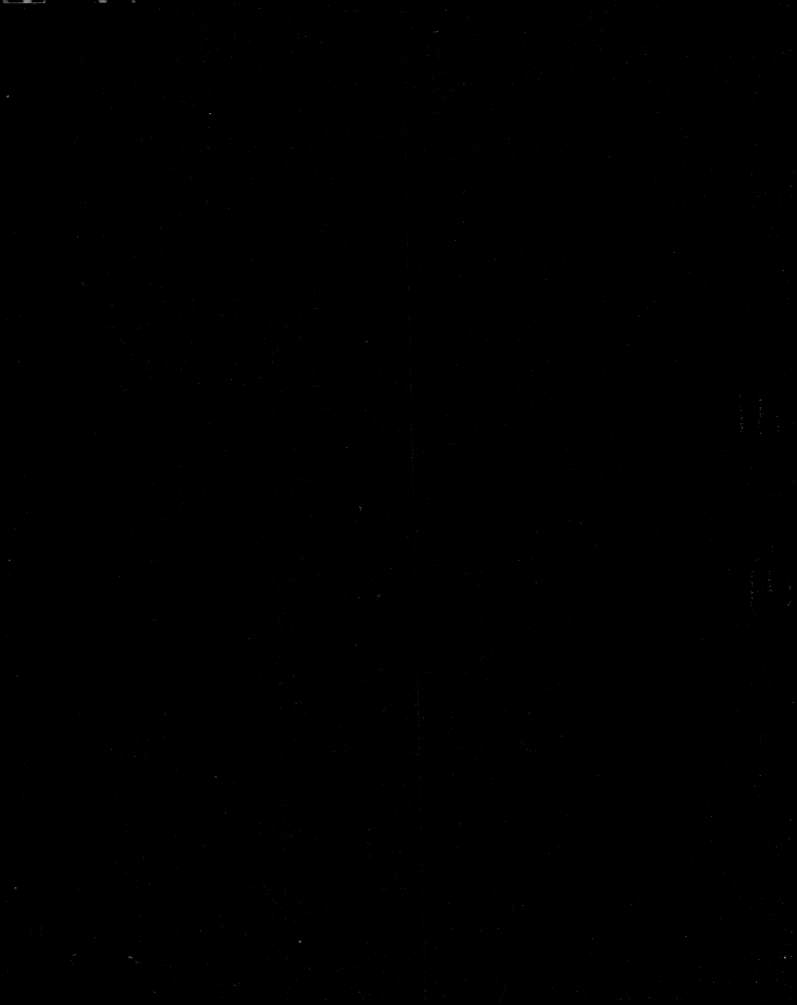

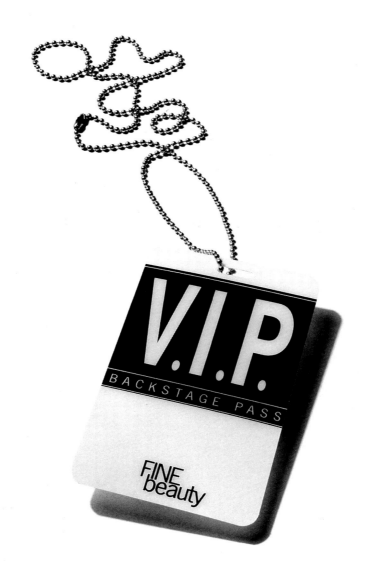

STARGAZING

When they coined the phrase "sugar and spice and every-thing nice," they must've had Tyra in mind. In a business where friendships are few and far between, I'm proud to call her a real friend. We met as both of our careers were blossoming, and grew up in this crazed business together. Tyra, blessed with brains and body (and what a body it is ☺), has definitely made her mark in the industry. Whether she's breaking down color barriers by being the first African-American model to grace the cover of Sports Illustrated, or mentoring inner-city youth, she's always poised and professional.

Tyra possesses a naturally sun-kissed complexion that's brought to life with golden glosses, apricot-colored blushers, and shimmery bronzers. Once they're applied she's immediately transformed into a gilded goddess.

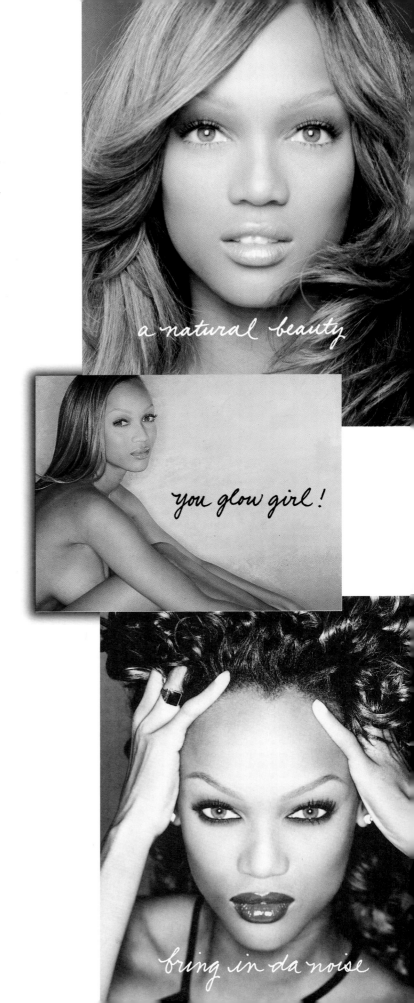

a natural beauty

you glow girl!

bring in da noise

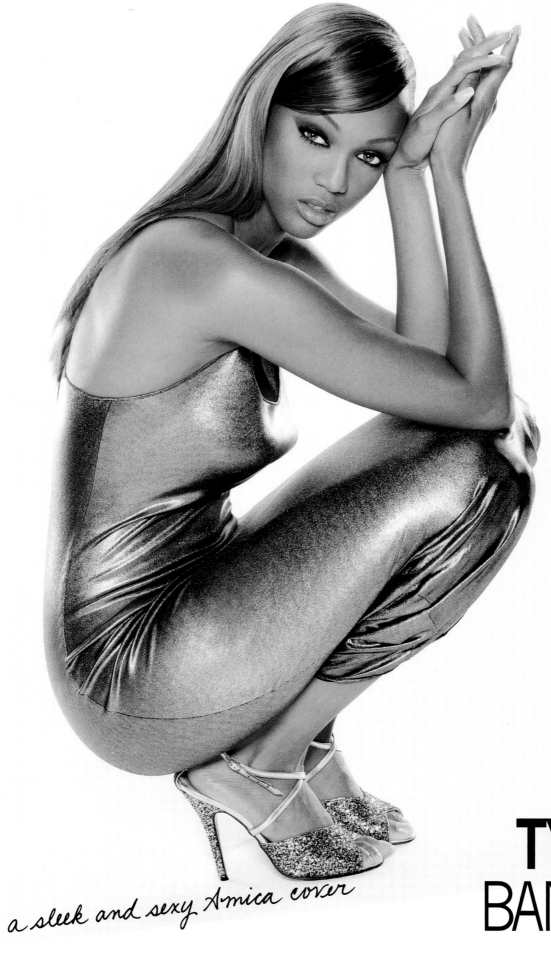

a sleek and sexy Amica cover

TYRA BANKS

One day, to my surprise, Patti called saying she was in a pinch. Her regular makeup artist wasn't available. She thought she'd give me a try. It ended up an evening of firsts for both of us — my first celebrity client and her first Grammy Award. Now, years later, we're still a winning team. She's remarkably like her stage persona; what you see is what you get. And she's not "just" the dynamic songstress known to bring down the house with a single note; she's a humanitarian with a heart, supporting causes like breast cancer awareness and AIDS research. She's been like a mother to me and has inducted me into her "family of many."

Patti's look is packed with star appeal, and that includes a great pair of lashes. If you've ever been to one of her concerts you might have taken one home as a souvenir, since she's famous for plucking them off midsong!

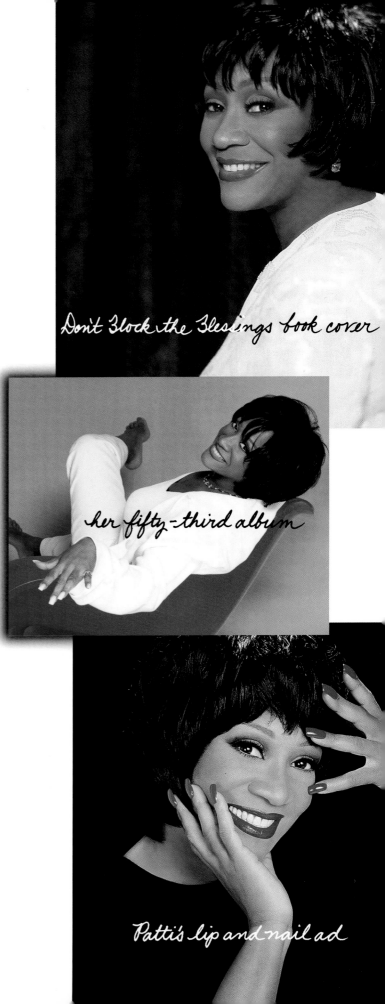

Don't Block the Blessings book cover

her fifty-third album

Patti's lip and nail ad

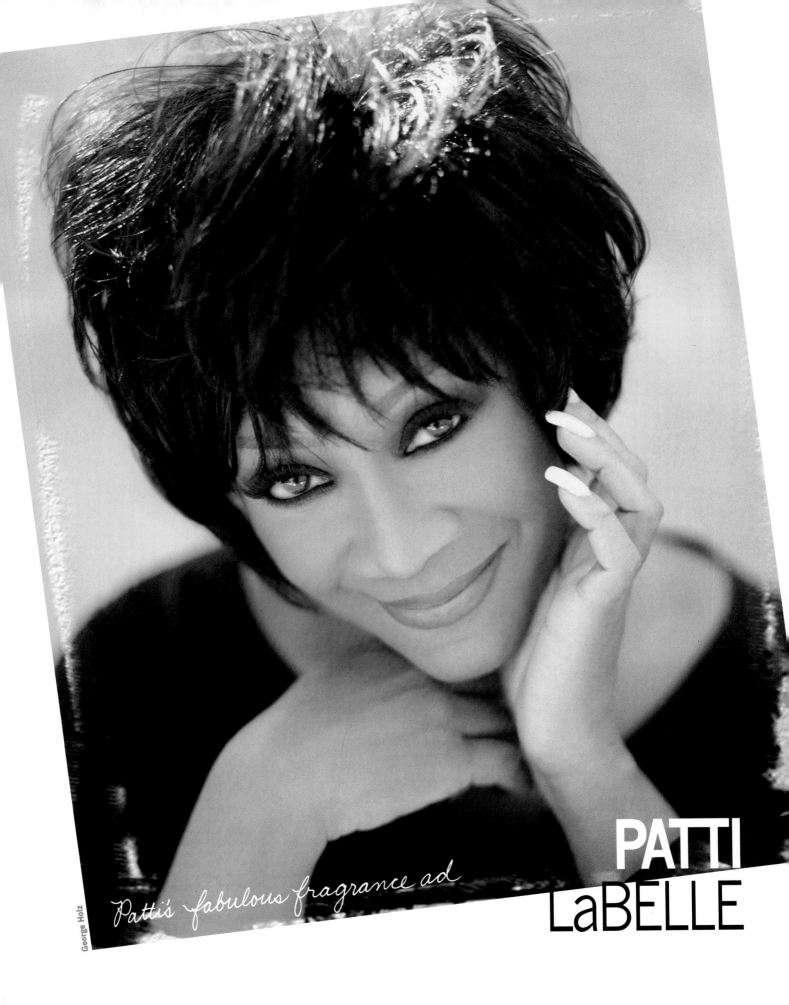

Patti's fabulous fragrance ad

PATTI LaBELLE

George Holz

I've admired Vanessa from the moment she was crowned Miss America. Gorgeous, poised, intelligent, and a host of other adjectives come to mind when describing her. Many people have asked me what she's like in real life. What I'm struck by is Vanessa as a mother: I've never seen a more caring parent. Whether appearing on the silver screen or a Broadway stage, or cutting her latest album, Vanessa always makes time for her children. Indeed, you might catch her at a drive-thru window of McDonald's picking up Happy Meals for her little ones. My hat's off to any entertainer who can put family above business as well as she does.

Vanessa enjoys the drama of a smoky lid. Neutral colors from warm beiges to chocolate browns are great for day, but our favorites are evening shades such as deep bronzes, dusky grays, and shimmering blues. Either is a knockout when paired with a nude, glossy mouth.

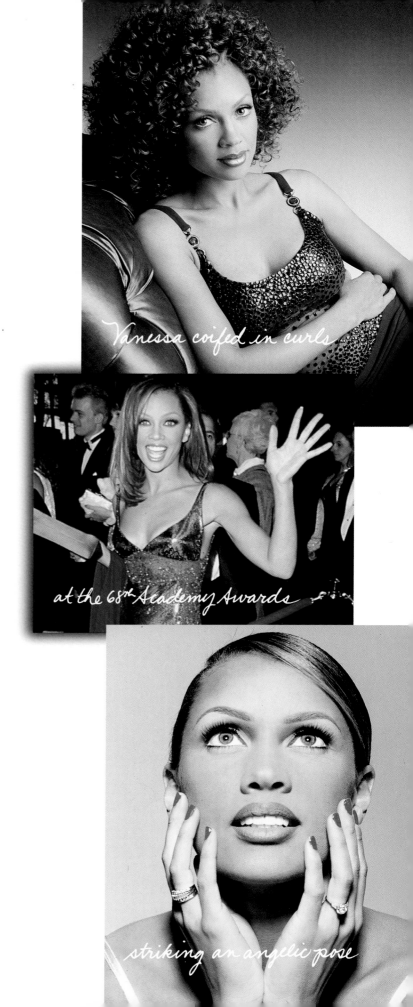

Vanessa coifed in curls

at the 68th Academy Awards

striking an angelic pose

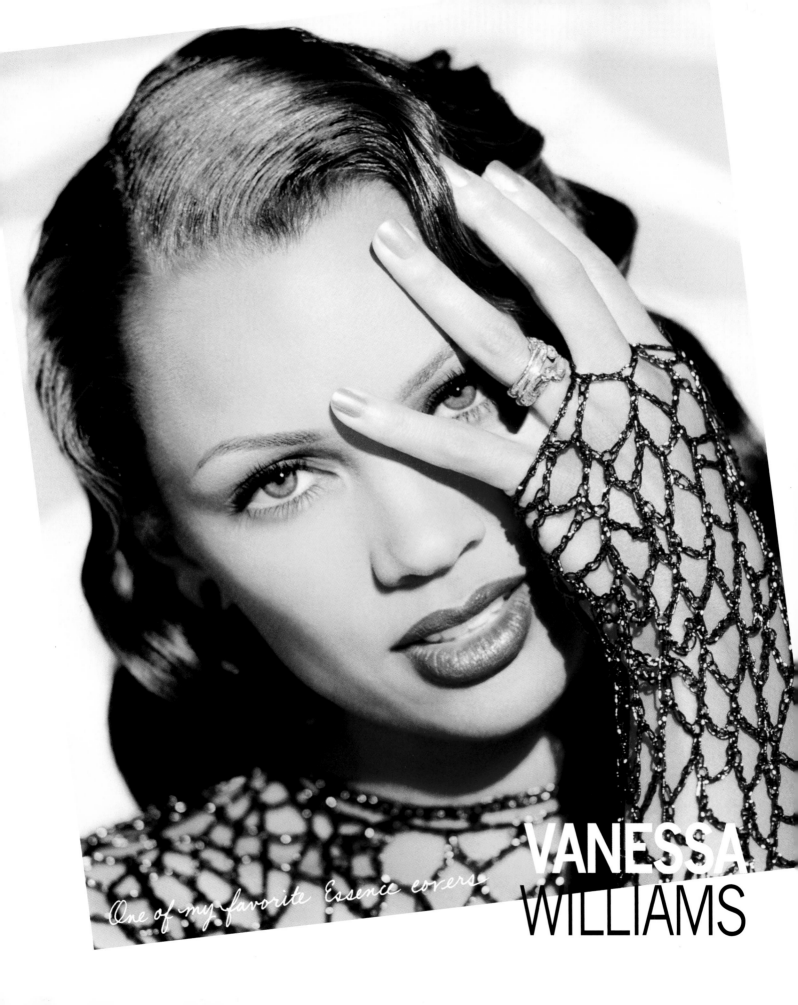

One of my favorite Essence covers

VANESSA WILLIAMS

I began working with Mary on the video for her single "Real Love." Since her first release had soared to the top of the charts, they called in the top guns to create a winning look. I was fortunate enough to be part of the ammunition. I really enjoy working with her. It was exciting to watch her meteoric rise to "Queen of Hip-Hop Soul" in the here-today, gone-tomorrow world of music.

Mary enjoys many different colors of lipstick, and her medium complexion accommodates a wide range of shades. I've applied colors from nude bronze to deep burgundy, and seen her sport edgier ones such as silver, blue, and even black! No matter how racy the shade, she wears it well.

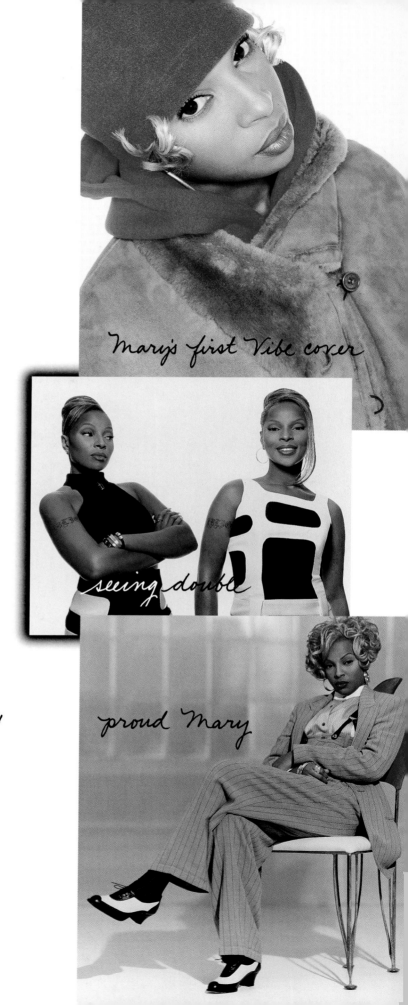

Mary's first Vibe cover

seeing double

proud Mary

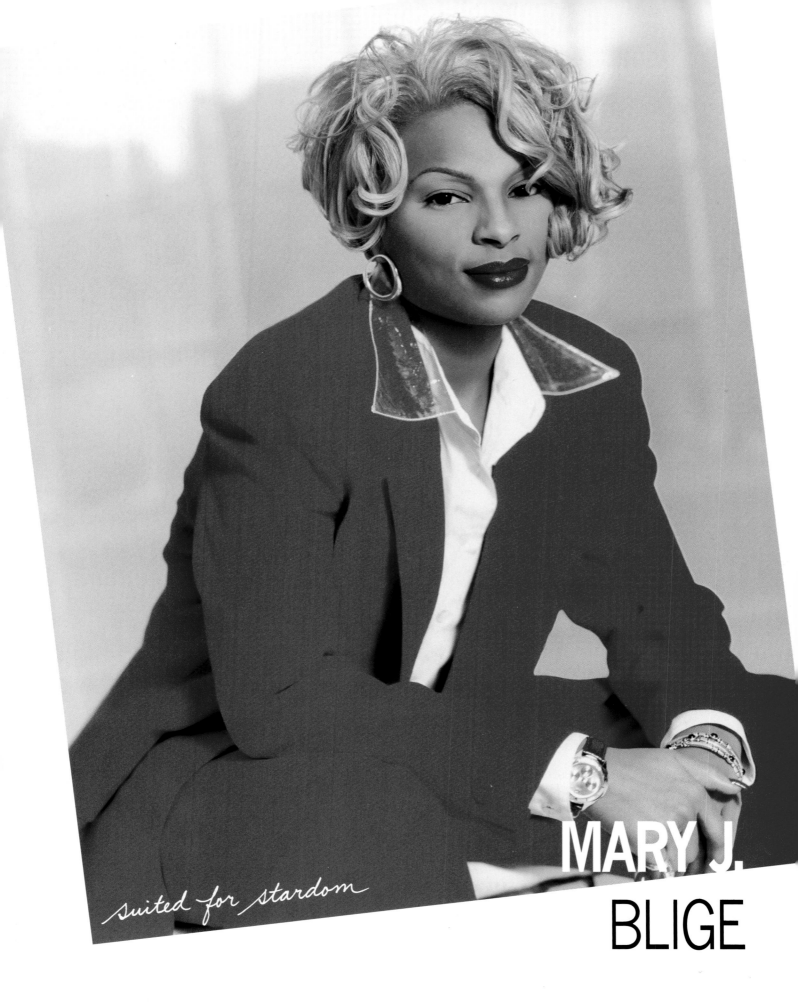

suited for stardom

MARY J.
BLIGE

Models are typically celebrated for their beauty, not their brains. Veronica gets major points for both. Aside from knowing how to strike a pose, she's fluent in two languages, is an award-winning journalist, and serves as a fashion correspondent for various media. Talk about a full plate! I've learned so much from her—everything from the importance of being on time for bookings to the need to keep a sharp eye on the dollars and cents. Thanks, V.

When Veronica first appeared on the scene, she was known as the girl with the thick, bushy eyebrows. I too am known for my eyebrows, or at least the ones I create. Over the years Veronica has allowed me to cut, bleach, and tweeze her eyebrows into a signature shape we both adore.

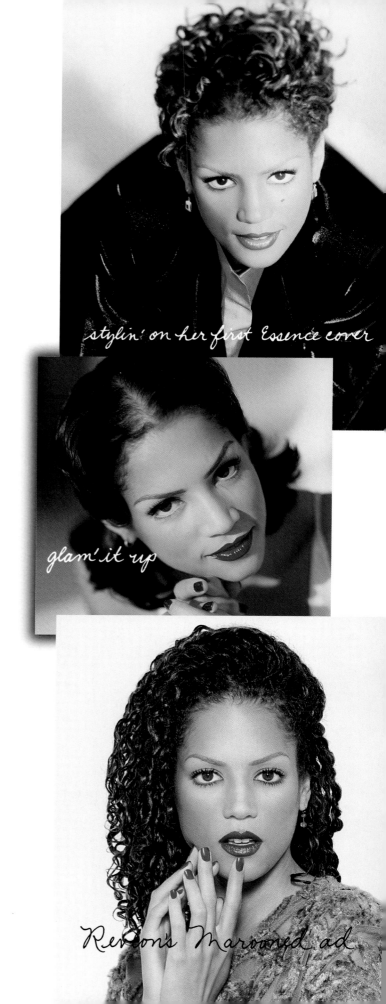

stylin' on her first Essence cover

glam' it up

Revlon's Marooned ad

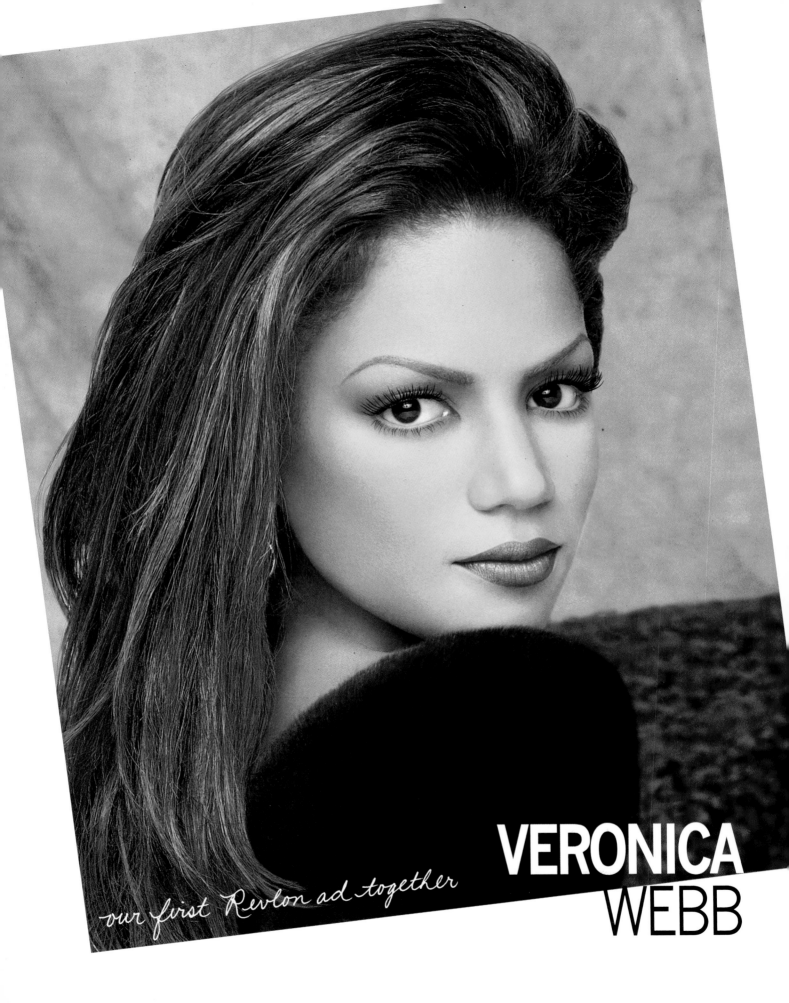

our first Revlon ad together

VERONICA
WEBB

Picture me standing behind the cosmetics counter. The phone rings. It's mega-model Naomi Campbell requesting me for a photo shoot. Wow! I had recently met her at a fashion show, while assisting top makeup artist Fran Cooper. This business isn't always kind to new kids on the block, so when I received Naomi's call I was shocked but delighted. After that she asked for me again on a number of high-profile assignments. She's always a pleasure to work with, because she gives you the freedom to create.

Naomi is the quintessential model. If you've ever seen her stalking the runways, then you know she thrives on dramatic change. Whether it's bleached brows, colored contacts, or an extreme hairstyle, Naomi knows how to work it.

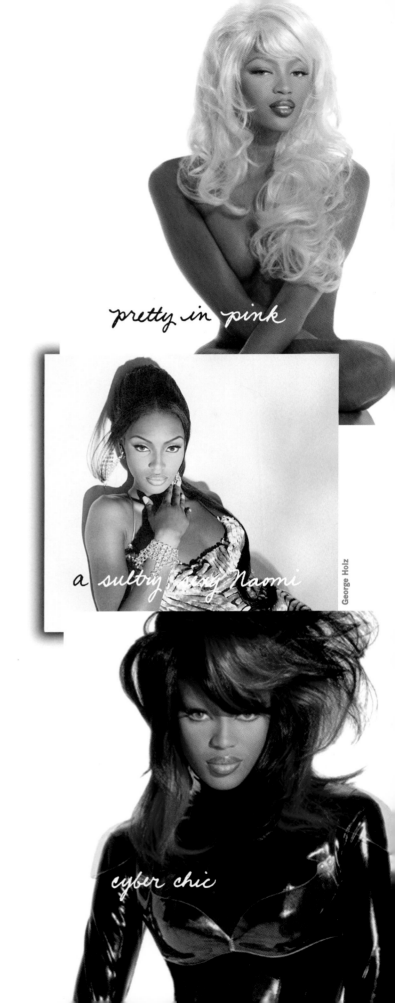

pretty in pink

a sultry, sexy Naomi

George Holz

cyber chic

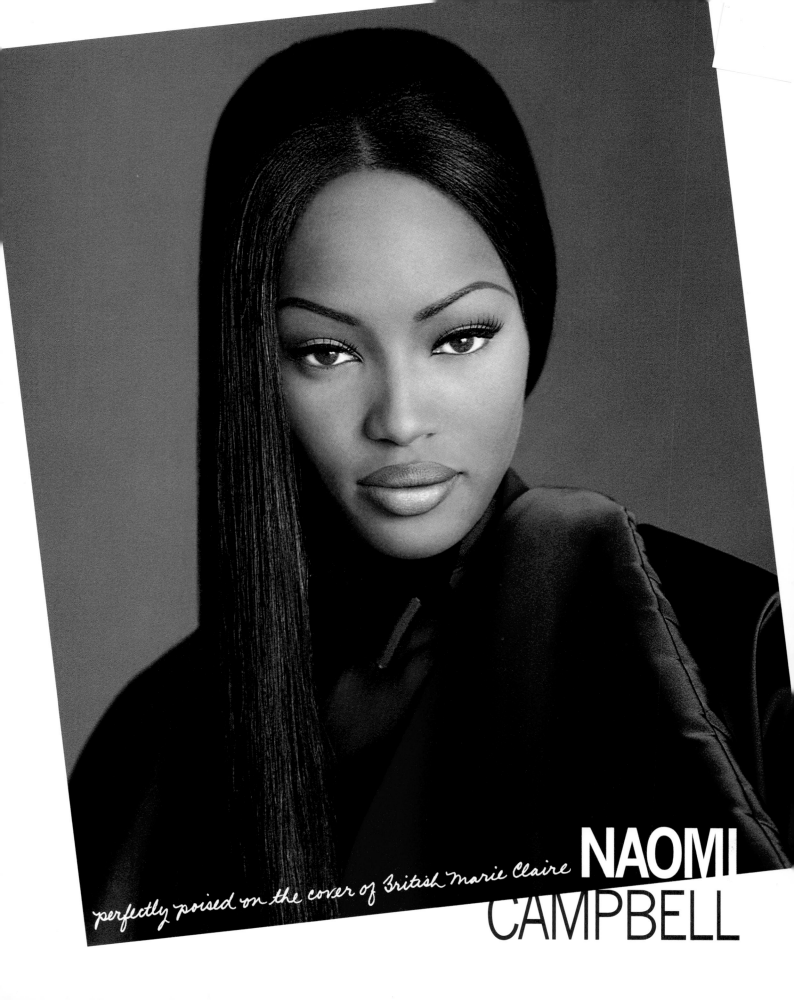

perfectly poised on the cover of British Marie Claire **NAOMI**
CAMPBELL

When I think back on my first impressions of Iman, visions of the Somalian siren gliding down the runway come to mind. In the world of fashion she is legendary. When I met her she immediately embraced me with a hug and kiss. I was thrilled to receive such a greeting. Working with her on several assignments has been a dream come true, and each photograph of her is always more amazing than the last.

Iman began her career at a time when it was hard to find foundations or powders to match her bronze complexion. Now, with more cosmetic lines to meet the needs of women of color (including her own wonderful brand), that's no longer a problem. In fact, cream foundation is one of my favorite products to use on Iman. It evens out her complexion to assure the flawless appearance she's known for.

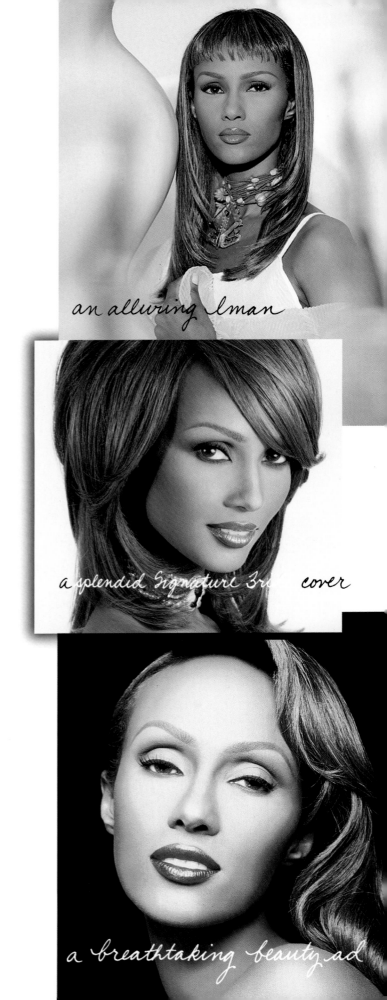

an alluring Iman

a splendid Signature Bride cover

a breathtaking beauty ad

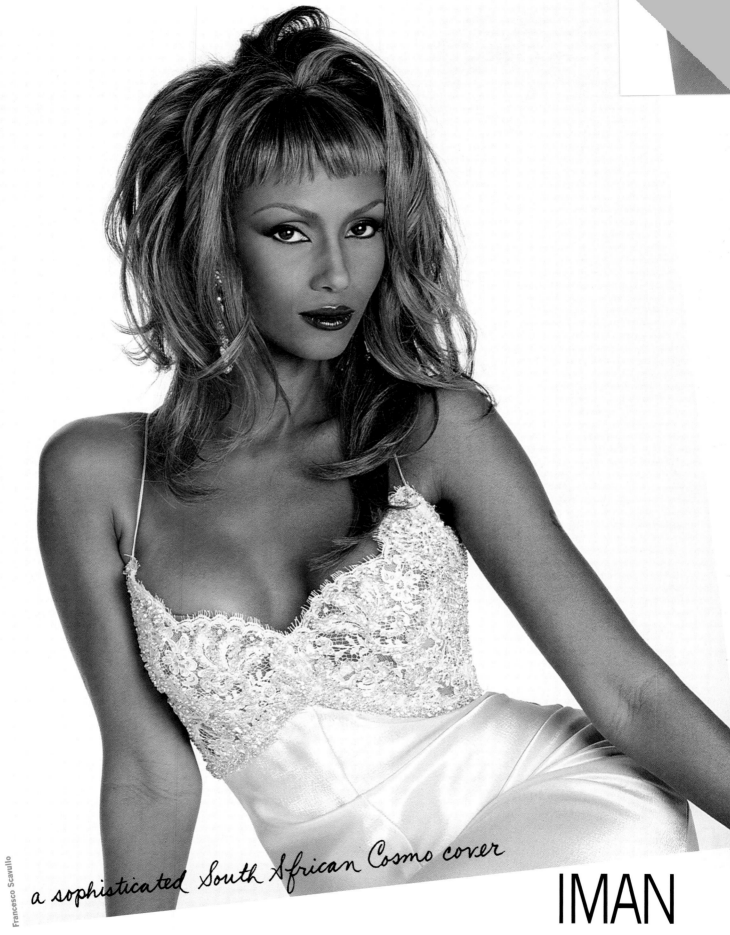

Francesco Scavullo

a sophisticated South African Cosmo cover

IMAN

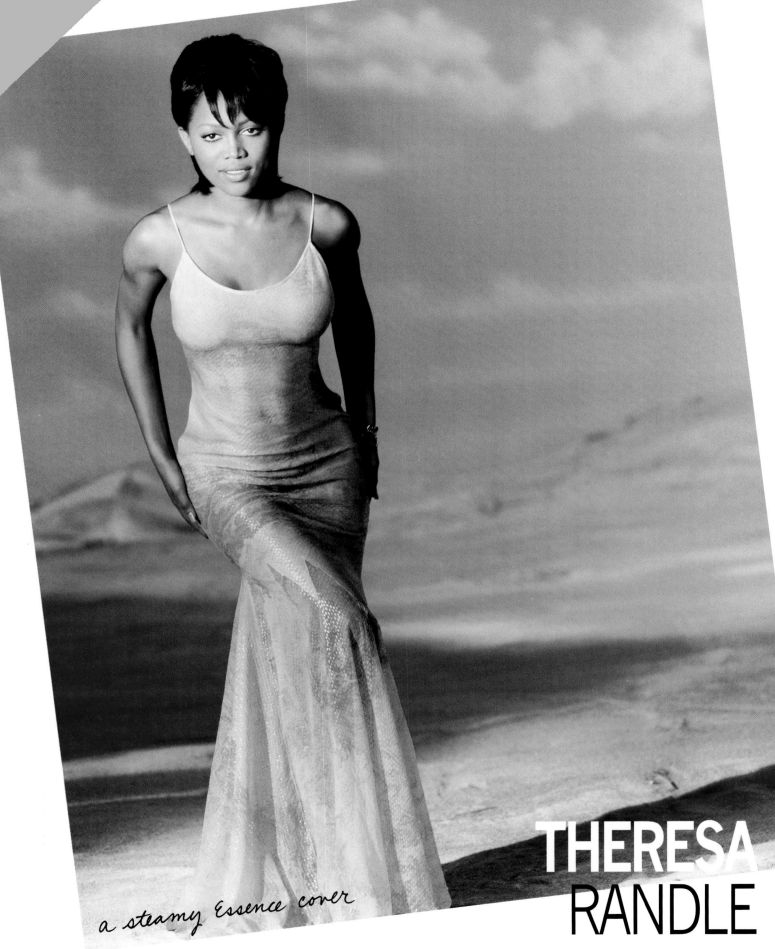

a steamy Essence cover

THERESA
RANDLE

I first worked with Theresa on an Essence cover shoot. She was fresh off the set of Spike Lee's Girl 6, where she had been the leading lady. The photographer's studio had been re-created to look like a beach, and I was charged with giving her a sultry siren-by-the-shore look. This didn't call for a face full of makeup, but rather a few coats of mascara and a dab of gloss across her lips to highlight her natural beauty. Theresa may be new to the big screen, but she knows exactly what to do in front of the camera.

"FINE IS A VISIONARY SOUL OF A WOMAN. NO FLAWS, NO ENDLESS

ARTIST; HE PAINTS THE
WITH HIM THERE ARE
PROBLEMS, JUST
POSSIBILITIES."

MIKKI TAYLOR,
BEAUTY AND COVER EDITOR,
ESSENCE

fine (fin), adj. 1. free from impurity. 2. superior in quality; of high or highest grade; excellent. 3. highly accomplished

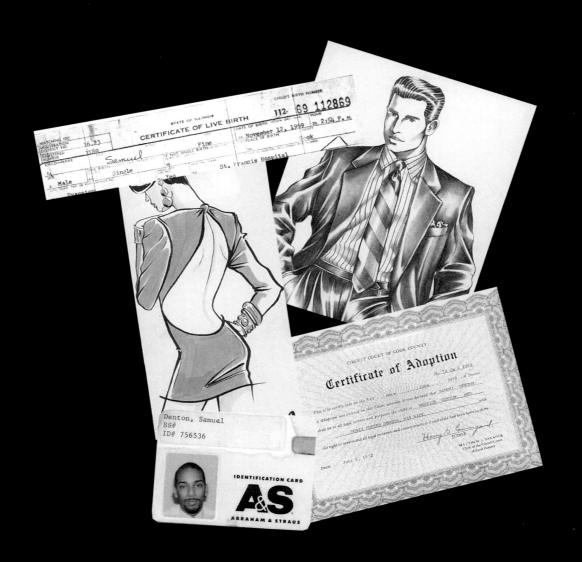

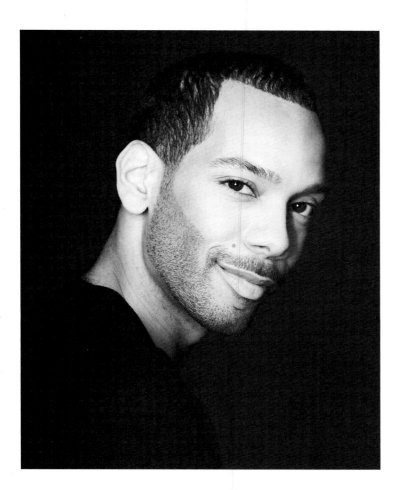

SAM FINE MAKEUP ARTIST

WHEN PEOPLE

ASK HOW I GOT STARTED

in the beauty biz, I usually give them the abbreviated version: I came to New York from Chicago with my sights set on becoming a fashion illustrator, the person who does the fashion sketches in newspapers and magazines. To support myself, I worked at a cosmetics counter in a department store, and I wound up becoming a makeup artist. Of course it wasn't that cut-and-dried. (Few things in life are.) Becoming a makeup artist was not my lifelong goal. I resisted it for a long time, until I realized how creatively satisfying it could be. Before I introduce you to the top people in beauty, fashion, and entertainment, I'd like to give you the unabridged version of how I came to be.

I was born in 1969 in Evanston, Illinois. Many people assume my name is made up, but Samuel Fine is my given name, as you can see from my birth certificate reproduced on the previous spread. When I was six months old, I was adopted into the loving family of Doris and Maurice Denton. There I became baby brother to Tracey, Kim, and Kina. Sometimes people ask me what it's like to be adopted, and all I can say is, "I don't know." For as long as I can remember, the family that celebrated my birthdays, the parents who taught me to ride a bicycle and took me to school every morning, were the only family I knew. From the moment my mom and dad adopted me, they loved me as if I were their own. I never felt that I wasn't an original member of the family.

As a child I was big on self-expression, dancing around and hamming it up every chance I got. But my real strength was my artistic ability. I liked to draw, and I was pretty good at it. It was an activity that my friends and I enjoyed the same way kids today enjoy video games: it was simply something fun to do. At the time it never dawned on me that it was a special talent that I would "draw" upon later in life. I first realized it was a special gift at Percy L. Julian High School, and I became much more serious about developing my skills. I concentrated on art and spent my spare time hanging out with the art teachers. I breezed through art classes, usually finishing my projects before everyone else. Then, restless and bored, I would devote the remainder of the period to harassing my classmates, which usually resulted in my getting in trouble and receiving low grades. When I wasn't being class clown, I was artist in chief of the school newspaper and yearbook. This position helped me develop my leadership abilities. At events like homecoming, football games, and school dances, I always contributed my artistic flair to the banners and posters that decorated our school. I began entering city- and statewide art contests, and winning. The prizes weren't big, but I thrived on the competition and on the recognition I received.

During my junior year one of my favorite art teachers recommended that I apply for a scholarship for a summer program at the Art Institute of Chicago. I did, and to my surprise I was accepted.

Attending this prestigious institution, even for just a summer, was a dream come true. My artistic abilities were taken to the next level, and it was here that I met a fashion illustration instructor, Craig "Rex" Perry, who would make an indelible mark on my life. Not only was he established in the industry, he was a profound teacher. He was one of my first mentors, and is an embodiment of the adage "Each one teach one." He took me under his wing, inviting me to sit in on other art classes, and challenged me to envision myself as a successful artist. I was so inspired by what I learned that summer that I began assembling my portfolio. I was on my way to becoming a fashion illustrator.

Trying to stay inspired back in high school, though, was a different story. I was a bright young man, but I did not have the same passion for other subjects that I had for art. During my senior year I cut classes, and for this I was suspended. At about the same time, I saw a newspaper ad seeking models for an upcoming hair show. With some free time on my hands, I decided to put it to use. I went to the casting and was selected as a model. There I met a designer who would become one of my best friends and yet another professional influence. Through him I was able to witness the activities of a young entrepreneur firsthand. Like my illustration instructor, he encouraged me, inspired me, and helped me realize my career potential.

I *barely* made it out of high school, but I made it. After I graduated, my designer friend decided to relocate to New York and asked if I wanted to come along for the ride. I didn't need much persuading. New York was to fashion what Hollywood was to movies. Like many creative types drawn to the Big Apple, we saw it as an opportunity to make it big and leave our mark in the fashion world. So in the fall of 1989, we packed our bags and headed east to find our fortune. Our new address, however, was far from Park Avenue. It was more like Hackensack, New Jersey, forty-five minutes from New York City. So much for taking the city by storm.

My days consisted of traveling thirty minutes by bus and reporting to my job as a salesperson at a department store, where I worked as holiday help. A friend introduced me to someone at a cosmetics line who needed a free-lance makeup artist. Though I didn't have any cosmetics experience to speak of, I had always watched my mother and three sisters making up. Besides, I had an art background, and through fashion illustration I had become familiar with some of the latest beauty trends. So I figured, Why not? If nothing else, it was a way for me to increase my meager earnings. I started by free-lancing on weekends. Unfortunately, even the two gigs I got weren't enough to help me make ends meet. After three months I was headed back to Chicago. Fortunately, the cosmetics company I had worked for was able to transfer me there, and as luck would have it, a year or so later my employers suggested I interview for a position in—where else?—New York! The company sent me a train ticket for the twenty-two-hour ride, and the trip was worth every minute. I got the job, and a second chance to realize my dreams.

In those early days of my career, I kept having what I call "meetings of kinship"—connections with good-hearted people who befriended and believed in me, and who were always willing to lend a helping hand. Joseph Hampton, for instance, played a major role in helping mold my career. An established makeup pro, he encouraged me in my fashion illustration pursuits, and later in my ambitions as a professional makeup artist. He coached me in the art of makeup and showed me the ropes of this sometimes fickle and demanding business.

With the support and guidance I'd received over the years, I soon felt confident enough to sample what the cosmetics industry had to offer. But before leaving my secure surroundings altogether, I invested my days off testing with photographers and assisting any makeup artist who would have me. My work as an assistant led to assignments at the New York collections, the showcase for America's top designers. And it was here that I met the model who would give me the chance of a lifetime: Naomi Campbell. After watching me shape brows and line lips backstage, she requested my services for an upcoming photo shoot. This was the first of many important bookings we would share. I was off to an exciting start. I met other supermodels and celebrities who would soon call upon my services. The life I had only dreamt of was becoming a reality.

When I look back, it's hard for me to believe I ever had a second thought about becoming a makeup artist. Reflecting on my life, and all the twists and turns it has taken, I feel blessed that I'm able to earn a living in a profession I enjoy. As you've just read, the making of my career was hardly a solo act. My success is due to many: parents who raised me, friends who encouraged me, and clients who respected my talent. While pursuing my career, I've had the pleasure of working with some of the most creative and talented people in beauty, fashion, and entertainment. Most are young, all are black, and their talent and wisdom abound. I thought it would be nice for you to meet them, and hear how they came to be the professionals they are today. They are living proof that with a head full of dreams, and a dose of determination, anything is possible. May their experiences inspire you to dream and motivate you to grow.

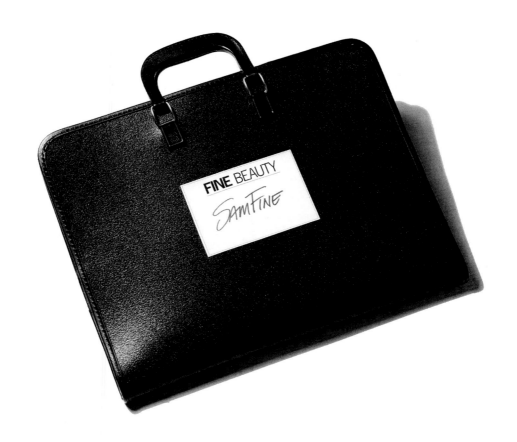

FINE FRIENDS

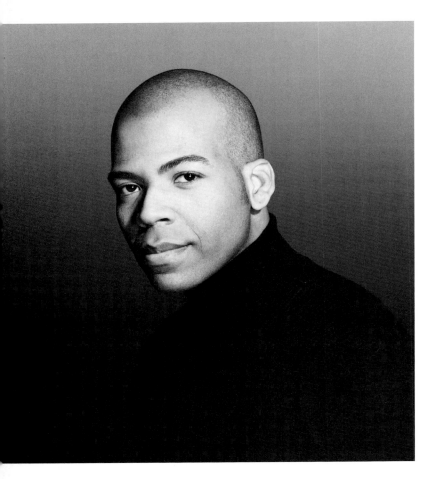

LLOYD BOSTON ART DIRECTOR

When sportswear designer Tommy Hilfiger first met Lloyd Boston at an in-store appearance, it was apparent that the Morehouse College sophomore had more on his mind than getting his promotional duffel bag autographed. Hilfiger was so impressed with what this aspiring young graphic artist had to say that he offered him an internship, on the spot. For Lloyd it was the first rung on a ladder of successes that would include becoming the company's first graphic designer, its director of graphic design two years later, and art director two years after that. (Twos haven't been terrible for Lloyd at all.) In his six years at Tommy Hilfiger this New Brunswick, New Jersey, native has played an integral role in all things creative, from advertising and promotion to fashion direction for runway shows. Just think: All this experience under his belt, and he's not even thirty!

HOW I GOT STARTED: By taking a non-paying position as a graphics intern at Tommy Hilfiger. It allowed me to see up close how design was done at a major Seventh Avenue fashion firm.

MY FIRST BIG BREAK: Meeting Tommy Hilfiger.

MY ADVICE TO OTHERS: To get your foot in the door, take any job that will have you anywhere near an art director—be it gofer, stylist, photographer's assistant, or intern—and begin to build a book of things that you've had a hand in. That book will be your calling card for other jobs. Once you're in, maintain a balance among the administrative, creative, and technical aspects

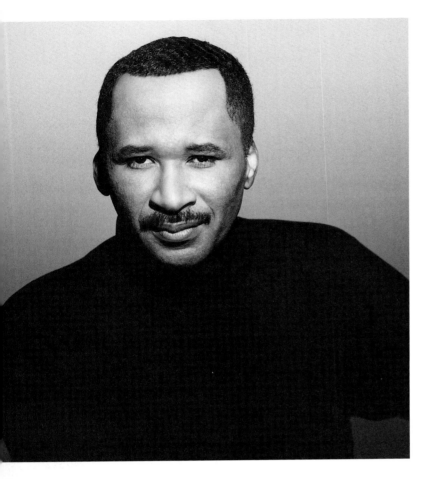

ANGELO ELERBEE PUBLICIST

It takes more than raw talent to make it in the music industry. Presentation is everything! That's why when record company executives need to smooth out the rough edges of their rising stars, they send them straight to Angelo Elerbee, founder and CEO of the Double Xxposure artist management and development firm. Inspired by Motown's in-house "charm school," the rigorous tutelage Berry Gordy provided for his artists back in the day, Angelo instructs artists on business skills, interview techniques, and the proper social graces needed to sustain them long after their recording is released. Shabba Ranks and Patra are just two of the names on Angelo's extensive roster, but the crowning achievement of his decade in business is the transformation of singer Mary J. Blige's 'round-the-way tough-girl image into that of the cool, urban R&B diva she is now. 'Nuff said.

HOW I GOT STARTED: I got my first
taste of publicity representing R&B artist Mtume, of the hit record "Juicy Fruit," and various artists on the New York club music scene, like Jocelyn Brown, Jomanda, and Sybil. I then went to work at Chrysalis Records, where I headed the publicity department. After learning the ropes of record industry PR, I was convinced I could do it on my own. I left to start Double Xxposure.

MY FIRST BIG BREAK: Becoming
Mtume's publicist. It was baptism by fire, but with his encouragement and support I quickly learned the ins and outs of the music industry.

MY ADVICE TO OTHERS: Becoming a
media sponge is key to making it in PR, because you've got to keep your finger on the pulse of what's happening in order to best help your clients. Read everything from newspapers to trade magazines, watch television, and go to movies, plays, and concerts. You'll be informed and inspired.

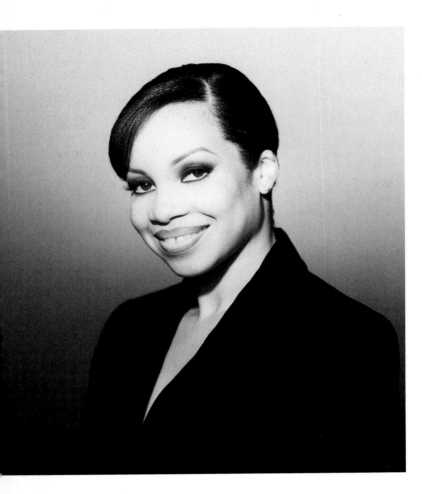

JERRI BACCUS GLOVER
MARKETING DIRECTOR

In the multibillion-dollar cosmetics industry, it's not enough simply to make pretty-colored lipstick—you have to be able to market products so that they sell, and sell well. That's Jerri Baccus Glover's job at Revlon. During her eighteen years there, the Cleveland native has played an integral role in the design and development of some of the company's top consumer and professional sellers, including ColorStyle, one of the most extensive makeup lines designed for women of color. And in a bold, progressive move, Jerri signed Veronica Webb to represent ColorStyle, making her the first African-American spokesmodel for a major cosmetics line. When the consumer demand for professional makeup lines began to grow, Jerri immediately recognized this trend and was visionary in the development of Revlon Professional (better known as R Pro), a forward line of makeup inspired by the products professional makeup artists use. So the next time you discover that perfect shade of lipstick, or find yourself admiring an attractive compact or struck by a model in an advertisement, know that for Jerri these results are all in a day's work.

HOW I GOT STARTED:

I worked as a dietitian in a hospital after graduating from Kent State University, but after six months on the job I realized it was not what I wanted to do. Shortly after, I landed a job in the sales division of Revlon's Cleveland offices.

MY FIRST BIG BREAK:

My promotion to Revlon's New York office was a breakthrough for me because it allowed me eventually to make the transition from sales to marketing. Marketing offered more opportunities for the kind of creativity I craved.

MY ADVICE TO OTHERS:

Don't settle for an occupation you no longer enjoy just because you majored in a related field. Earning a degree is only the beginning. It's what you do with it that makes the difference. Find a way to parlay your skills in a field that you do like. If it's marketing, determine which areas and companies interest you. Marketing is different from industry to industry. The principles are the same, but how you approach it can vary. Once you get a job treat it like a classroom, and never stop learning.

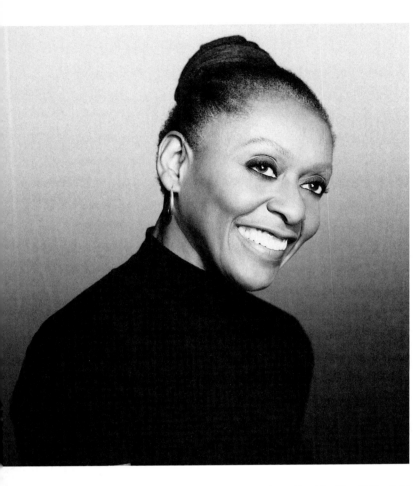

BETHANN HARDISON
TALENT MANAGER

In recent years, Bethann Hardison has gained a rep for helping establish the stellar careers of some very talented men, first as model/muse to the late, great designer Willi Smith, then as mother/manager to actor Kadeem Hardison, and more recently as the motherly manager to mega male model Tyson Beckford, who, like a son, gives her props every chance he gets. During the seventies, she made a name for herself as a legendary black model, regularly sparking the runways at European fashion shows. Accomplishments like these are just a few of the feathers in the cap of this native New Yorker and Seventh Avenue veteran. Don't ask her what she's done, ask her what she hasn't. From her humble beginnings as a bookkeeper, to more prestigious positions with Stephen Burrows, Valentino, and other designers, to running her own modeling agency, Bethann has worked Fashion Avenue like no other and has lived to tell about it.

HOW I GOT STARTED: Frances Grill, the founder of Click Model Management, asked me to come work for her soon after she opened shop. Even though I'd never booked models before, I knew how to do a lot of different things, and when you know how to do a lot of different things you can lend your expertise to any situation.

MY FIRST BIG BREAK: In the broadest sense of the term, I don't think my big break has happened yet. I'm still looking, and forever ambitious. As far as what I am currently doing, my break came when I took the advice of a few of the models I represented and opened my own agency.

MY ADVICE TO OTHERS: There's no formula to managing—I can't tell you how to do it in three easy steps. It's sort of like picking up whatever falls on the floor. You have to be willing and able to do everything you can to get things done, and maintain a sense of integrity through it all.

OSCAR JAMES HAIRSTYLIST

Vanessa Williams, Iman, Veronica Webb, and Tyra Banks all trust their tresses to hairstylist extraordinaire Oscar James. That's because the coifs he creates for them say high style. For Oscar, it's all in a day's work. He's been fiddlin' with hair ever since he was a boy in Florence, South Carolina, where he studied cosmetology in high school and worked part-time at a salon. A few years after graduating, with diploma and cosmetology license in hand, Oscar moved to New York City to broaden his creative horizons. He landed a gig at a highly visible midtown salon, where he became so popular he was scheduled with appointments for months in advance. With a reputation this hot, it was only a matter of time before he was scooped up by the celebrity set to become the star hairstylist he is today.

HOW I GOT STARTED: From a young age I gravitated to hairstyling like a magnet. I worked on anyone who would let me. I'd give my cousins corn rows, and set my mother's hair in curlers every night, then style it in the morning.

MY FIRST BIG BREAK: Being called on to style Vanessa Williams's hair for a video.

MY ADVICE TO OTHERS: Put God first in all that you do. Establish yourself at a salon, prefer-ably one where a lot of people will see your work, and practice your craft. Maintain an even temperament (this always helps when you're working with a lot of different personalities). Most of all, don't lose sight of your reg-ular clientele, even while working the celebrity circuit; your regulars help you stay grounded in this sometimes unpredictable industry.

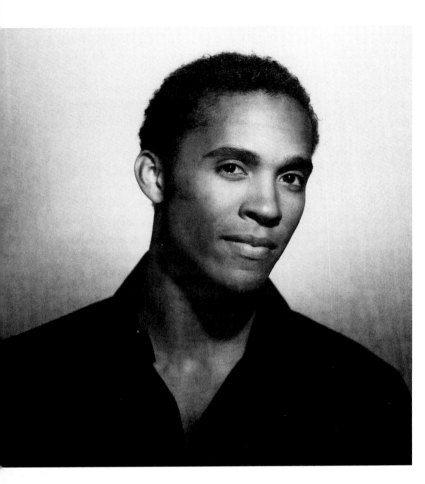

RON NORSWORTHY
SET DESIGNER

With paint, props, and plenty of artistic vision, Ron Norsworthy has created sets for a number of commercials and films. But set design for music videos is where this Iowa native has made his mark. He gave Busta Rhymes a bright monochromatic edge in his "Woo-Hah!!" video by crafting wild and lively scenes to match the rapper's wild and lively wardrobe; he also helped Toni Braxton come across as a vulnerable chanteuse in her video for "I Don't Wan't To" by constructing the minimalist space she performs in. I have actually seen him work wonders transforming an empty soundstage into what appeared to be a fully stocked supermarket aisle, for Maxi Priest's "That Girl" video. When Ron lets his imagination rip, watch out!

HOW I GOT STARTED: I was an architect. I fell into set design when friends who were in film school started asking me to design the sets for their student projects. As their careers took off in film and video, so did mine.

MY FIRST BIG BREAK: Being asked by Spike Lee to serve as an art director on *Crooklyn,* where I got to work with Wynn Thomas, a production designer I very much admire.

MY ADVICE TO OTHERS: Having a background in architecture, fine arts, and decorative arts is crucial in succeeding as a cinematic production designer. Architecture gives you a keen understanding of how space is utilized, while knowledge of fine and decorative arts helps you develop a sense of aesthetics. A knowledge of carpentry also helps, but it is absolutely essential that you know how to draw, so that you can present your ideas pictorially, which is the first step in set design.

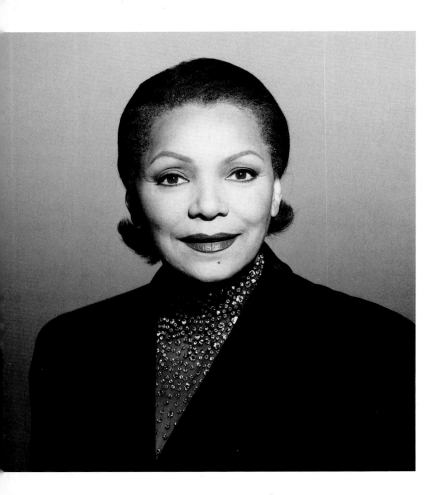

AUDREY SMALTZ
BACKSTAGE FASHION PRODUCER

When top designers Donna Karan, Bill Blass, and Vera Wang need backstage help with their fashion shows, who they gonna call? None other than Audrey Smaltz and her ultra-efficient Ground Crew. The team, which she founded, is responsible for backstage management, which includes dressing models to designers' specifications and seeing to it that they walk down the runway on cue—and that's not easy, when you consider how backstage at a fashion show can be compared to a landing strip at O'Hare: hectic! But Audrey is a pro. She spent her formative years working a few runways herself, when Iman was probably just learning how to walk and Naomi Campbell wasn't even a twinkle in her parents' eyes. And for the better part of the seventies, hers was the voice for the *Ebony* Fashion Fair, that legendary touring fashion show sponsored by *Ebony* magazine, where most of us got our first glimpse of high fashion in motion. In short, Audrey knows fashion like no other, and that's what keeps those designers calling.

HOW I GOT STARTED:

During my stint with *Ebony,* I noticed that a lot of designers used people to dress their models. I thought that providing designers with a crew of people who specialized in just this would be a great service, so I looked to establish my own business. I hand-delivered about a hundred letters to various Seventh Avenue designers describing my service and got responses from only three. But I knew that this was something they needed, whether or not they realized it, and I persevered.

MY FIRST BIG BREAK:

One of the three people who responded, at a French sportswear company, took me up on my offer. But there's really no such thing as your first big break—I've been preparing for this my whole life. I was in the right place at the right time, and they needed me.

MY ADVICE TO OTHERS:

When setting out to be in business for yourself, you have to be dedicated, prepared, and totally focused on what you do. Associate with people who are where you want to be, and stay clear of negative people; they will only bring you down. Most important, keep God in the center of your life and you won't have anything to worry about.

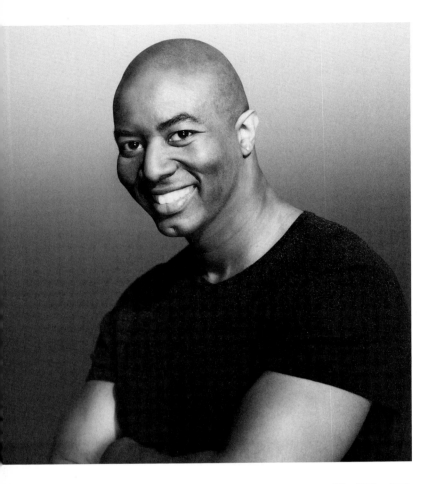

MATTHEW JORDAN SMITH
PHOTOGRAPHER

Picture this: A young boy growing up in Columbia, South Carolina, receives a camera as a gift. His father, an avid amateur photographer, shows him the basics of picture taking, and the boy is hooked. The family bathroom becomes his makeshift darkroom, and anything within focus of his viewfinder is fair game. Zoom forward: It's the nineties, and country boy has grown into city slicker, his work regularly gracing the covers of major publications and national ad campaigns. Through his lens he has gazed upon such stars as Oprah, Angela Bassett, Vanessa Williams, and Erykah Badu. In the brief six years that he has been taking pictures professionally, Matthew has reached career heights that most photographers only dream of. But what else would you expect from such a focused young man?

HOW I GOT STARTED: I loved photography from the minute I picked up my first camera. After high school I enrolled at the Art Institute of Atlanta with the intention of becoming a sports photographer. But after being exposed to fashion photography, I knew it was the field for me.

MY FIRST BIG BREAK: Shooting a fashion story and a celebrity profile for *Essence* magazine.

MY ADVICE TO OTHERS: Study magazines to familiarize yourself with the latest trends and techniques, as well as the photographers who are making it happen. Assist photographers who are doing the kind of work you want to do, and test with models, stylists, and hair and makeup people for practice and to build a portfolio.

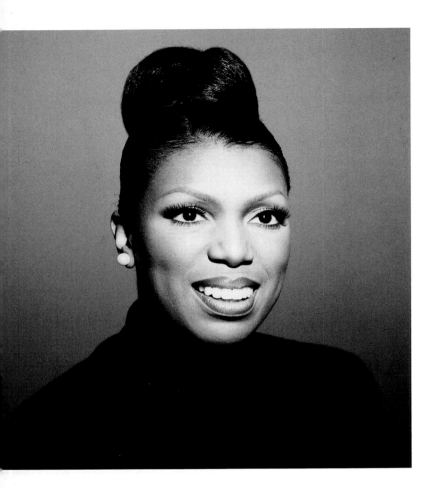

MIKKI TAYLOR
BEAUTY EDITOR

or more than a decade, Mikki Taylor, beauty and cover editor for *Essence* magazine, has shown us just how beautiful black can be. From the arresting images you see on the outside each month to the latest news on cosmetics hair care, and fragrances inside, Mikki gives sisters information and affirmation that is paralleled by no other major publication.

A native of Newark, New Jersey, Mikki has a knack for beauty that comes honestly. Her mother traveled the world as stylist to jazz legend Sarah Vaughan, then brought her know-how to the black women in her community by opening a hair salon, and Mikki likens what she does at *Essence* to what her mother did: helping black women celebrate their unique beauty and style.

HOW I GOT STARTED:
When I was a merchandise coordinator for Tahari, a manufacturer of career wear for women, I worked closely with the design team selecting textiles. It was the early eighties, and black women were entering the professional work force in a big way. In response to that, *Essence* offered fashion features showing women how to make clothes that reflected their style for work. When the magazine had an opening for an accessories and home sewing editor, people on its fashion team who knew me from Tahari encouraged me to apply, so I did.

MY FIRST BIG BREAK:
Breaks come to you mentally long before you reach any tangible opportunities—they're those moments when you first set out to reach your goal. My tangible break came when Susan Taylor made me beauty editor once she became editor in chief at *Essence*.

MY ADVICE TO OTHERS:
If you're interested in becoming a beauty editor, I would encourage you first to get the journalistic training you need. Then learn about the beauty business inside and out, past and present. Keep abreast of the latest trends and techniques as well as the companies driving them. Being informed will help you sail successfully in this industry.

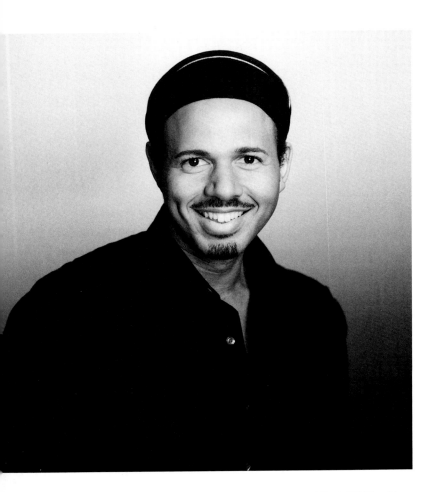

EMIL WILBEKIN
FASHION DIRECTOR

Where popular music and fashion intersect, you'll find Emil Wilbekin. As fashion director for *Vibe*, the monthly devoted to all things hip and urban, he gives the magazine visual flavor by producing its edgy covers and fashion pages as well as by making our favorite artists look like fashion plates. (Who could forget that fly spread he did featuring Foxy Brown, the Notorious B.I.G., Mary J. Blige, and other hip-hop and R&B greats dressed in designer gear and posed like characters in scenes from classic Hitchcock movies?) The fabulous pictures you see are the end result of the great lengths this Cincinnati native goes to: he shops around the world for the latest fashions, and assembles photographers, models, and hair and makeup artists for shoots, and sometimes just walks the streets of New York City to check the latest styles on the kids.

HOW I GOT STARTED:

After majoring in mass media in college, I worked as an editorial assistant at *Metropolitan Home* magazine and free-lanced as a fashion reporter for Associated Press and the *Chicago Tribune*. Later, after getting my master's in journalism, I was recommended for a position as an associate editor on the premiere issue of *Vibe*. Here I conceptualized ideas and wrote copy for the fashion section. When *Vibe* became a full-fledged monthly, I was responsible for producing celebrity photo sessions. Soon after, I was promoted to style editor and styled the photo shoots I planned. All of that prepared me for my current position as fashion director.

MY FIRST BIG BREAK:

The first photo shoot I styled for *Vibe* featuring Tyson Beckford.

MY ADVICE TO OTHERS:

Whatever field you're trying to get into, be it publishing or fashion, make sure you study it thoroughly. If you want to be a stylist, you should study the work of an established stylist. Assisting is a great way to learn the tricks of the trade.

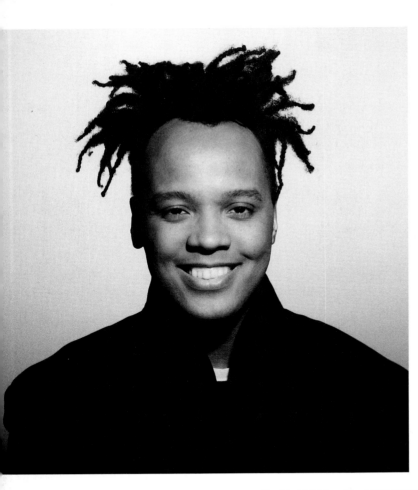

EDWARD WILKERSON
FASHION DESIGNER

Behind every successful clothing design house is a designer whose sole job is to execute the vision and philosophy of the house. Edward Wilkerson is one such designer. For more than a decade he's been at the drawing board at Donna Karan, where his tasteful approach and sense for spare yet sophisticated styling has helped make the label a household name among the fashionable set. For this talented native New Yorker, the position is par for the course. He made his debut in fashion designing for an accessories firm while still a student at the High School of Art and Design. And before Donna, he put in some time at two other big K's on Seventh Avenue: Calvin Klein and Anne Klein. Though Edward is a bona fide fashion industry veteran, having worked on many a collection, he still gets excited watching his chic designs parade down the runway each season, just as if it were his first.

HOW I GOT STARTED: I've been an artist since I was very young. Once I got to high school I progressed toward fashion and started designing.

MY FIRST BIG BREAK: Landing a job on the design team of Anne Klein.

MY ADVICE TO OTHERS: Immerse yourself in your craft. Study designers and the types of clothes they make, read fashion magazines, attend trunk shows at department stores. Practice drawing, sewing, draping, and any other skill that will help you in clothing design and construction. If you want to become a designer, you have to live it!

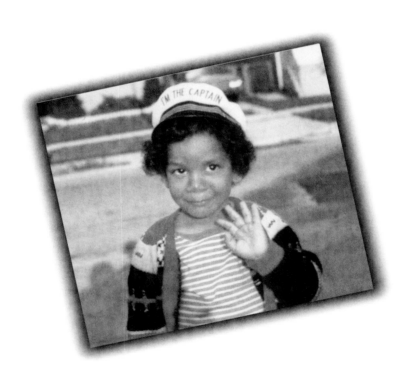

ACKNOWLEDGMENTS

I first thank God for bestowing such a talent upon me, and for placing so many dynamic individuals in my life.

My undying gratitude to Mom and Dad for opening their hearts and their home, raising me in love, and endlessly supporting my endeavors; to my sisters, Tracey, Kim, and Kina, for always taking care of their "baby brother"; and to my brothers-in-law, Joseph and James, who watch over them. I love you all!

Thank you, Veronica Webb, for a fabulous foreword, for friendship, and for your continued support.

My deep appreciation to Matthew Jordan Smith for donating week-days, weekends, and holidays to make this book its photographic best. Your contribution is priceless.

I thank Keith Major for finding the time to create the exquisite black-and-white photographs of models and other professionals featured in this book.

Thanks to Robert Tardio, who made each and every still-life shot come to life.

Many thanks to Lloyd Boston. As if he weren't busy enough with his own book, he found time to help me create a classic template that will excite for years to come.

Thank you, Julia Chance, for helping me express my thoughts and for giving our readers words of empowerment. You're so special!

Special thanks to my editor, Mary South, for believing in me and my vision. Your patience, understanding, and guidance were just what I needed.

To everyone at Riverhead, especially Bill Peabody, Claire Vaccaro, Ann Spinelli, Lisa Amoroso, Sarah Manges, and Anna Jardine, thanks for your tireless dedication and professionalism. Whew—we did it!

To another fabulous team of professionals—Marilyn Ducksworth, Matthew Snyder, Jason Weinberg, and Alise Konialian—thanks for putting the word out and making sure it appears in print and other media.

Thank you, Armstead and Patti Edwards, for taking me in as part of the family. Your support and understanding have helped make my career what it is today. Thanks to the team at PAZ Management: Fahja for her tireless assistance, and Art and Vance for all their hard work. Thanks also to my agent, Jean Owen, and her assistant, Mary Lou Bushi, for their support and patience throughout the years.

Thanks also to Mike Pietrangelo and Sharon Boone for taking a serious interest in me and recognizing what I have to contribute to the cosmetics industry.

To Tyra Banks, Naomi Campbell, Iman, Patti LaBelle, Brandy Norwood, Mikki Taylor, Veronica Webb, and Vanessa Williams, thanks for your heartfelt quotes and your support throughout my career. I am elated to have you as clients, and blessed to call you friends.

A super-special thanks to Lene Hall for gracing the cover of this tome. Your beauty radiates from within. And to the bevy of beauties —Cynthia Bailey, Wendy Brooks, Kishina Covington, Tammy Ford, Maureen Gallagher, Janine Green, Tia Holland, Gail O'Neill, Marie Powell, Sharon Russell, Tomiko, and Roshumba Williams—for their professionalism and devotion to this project. I owe you all!

I am extremely grateful to my makeover subjects—Donna McCoy, Sharon Miller, Marie Powell, Erana Stinson, and my mom, for allowing me to bleach, tweeze, powder, and paint them for hours. Thanks to Carolyn London for her contributions to the makeover chapter, and to RuPaul for taking time out of his hectic schedule and trusting me to help him make him look his best.

To the many talented photographers who graciously allowed me to use their brilliant work in this book—Miles Aldrige, Barron Claiborne, Patrick Demarchelier, Daniela Frederici, Steve Granitz, Hiromasa, George Holz, Christophe Jouany, Gideon Lewin, Keith Major, Elisabeth Novick, Michael O'Neill, Albert Sanchez, Francesco Scavullo, Matthew Jordan Smith, Michael Thompson, Nick Vaccaro, and Timothy White—thanks for always making my work look its absolute best. Thanks also to the many companies that gave permission to display shots from some of my favorite music videos and commercials.

Thanks to my "fine friends"—Lloyd Boston, Angelo Elerbee, Jerri Baccus Glover, Bethann Hardison, Oscar James, Ron Norsworthy, Audrey Smaltz, Matthew Jordan Smith, Mikki Taylor, Emil Wilbekin, and Edward Wilkerson—for making themselves available for interviews and portrait sittings. Your lives and experiences serve as an inspiration to all.

Thanks to the many hairstylists who coifed each model: Chuckie Amos, Mathu Anderson, Kelvin Brooks, Johnny Gentry, James Harris, Oscar James, Tony Marshall, and Annu Prestonia and Ruth Sinclair of Khamit Kinks New York City and Atlanta, respectively; to the clothes stylists who dressed the models: Sharon Miller, Donna McCoy, Elaine Wallace, and David Dalrymple for the House of Field; to the manicurist who sculpted each nail, Bernadette Thompson; and to Laura Mohberg, who assisted me through it all with a smile.

Thanks also to the wonderful staff at Montage Studio for accommodating my every photo shoot.

Thanks to Art Westphal and his team of many for their meticulous work; you've helped make beautiful images absolutely flawless.

A very special thanks to *all* my friends who bring joy and happiness into my life every day; and to Martin and Karen, Derwin, Kenya, Richard, Ty, Veronica, Dehaven, Erol, Danny, Gina, Matthew, Norma, Oscar, and Tony for putting up with me since the inception of this book. Without your constant support and encouragement, I could never have started or completed this project.

And the most heartfelt thanks to Joseph Michael Hampton, for taking me under his wing and teaching me to fly!

I also must express my appreciation to each and every person whose work is featured in this book; without you there would be no me.

If I were to list every person who aided in locating the perfect photo or video, in booking models and scheduling professionals, or in gathering approvals for all of the above, that would be a book in itself (trust me, I tried). I hope it will suffice for me to give one great big THANK YOU to you all! You helped make each image come to life.

Finally, I thank _____, because I'm sure I've
                       (YOUR NAME HERE)
forgotten someone.

CREDITS

all still-life photographs: Robert Tardio

pages 6, 16, 28-35, 54-61: Matthew Jordan Smith

pages 8, 36-45, 128-148: Keith Major

page 69: "Brokenhearted," courtesy Atlantic Records

page 71: "I Wanna Be Down," courtesy Atlantic Records

page 73: "Sentimental" and "Who Do U Love," courtesy Arista Records, Inc.

page 75: "Freek'n You," courtesy MCA Records

page 77: "Right Kinda Lover" and "When You Talk About Love," courtesy MCA Records

page 79: "Keep On, Keepin' On," courtesy Elektra Entertainment Group

pages 81, 83: Li'l Penny commercials, courtesy Nike, Inc.

page 85: "That Girl," courtesy Virgin Records

page 87

left: "Colors of the Wind" © 1995 Disney Entertainment, courtesy Disney Entertainment

right: "The Sweetest Days," courtesy Mercury Records

page 89: "Missing You," courtesy Atlantic Records

page 91: "Don't Want to Lose," courtesy Mercury Records

page 93: "Model Dave," courtesy Wendy's

page 98

top: Daniela Frederici for *YM*

center: Michael O'Neill, for *People* magazine, "50 Most Beautiful" issue

bottom: Matthew Jordan Smith for Ty Girl, Inc.

page 99: Christophe Jouany for *Amica*

page 100

top: Nick Vaccaro for *Don't Block the Blessings* book jacket, courtesy Riverhead Books

center: Albert Sanchez for *Flame* album cover, courtesy MCA Records

bottom: Gideon Lewin for Patti LaBelle Lip and Nail line, courtesy Johnson Products

page 101: © 1996 George Holz for Patti LaBelle Fragrance

page 102

top: Matthew Jordan Smith for *Essence*

center: Steve Granitz at the Academy Awards

bottom: Daniela Frederici, courtesy Mercury Records

page 103: Matthew Jordan Smith for *Essence*

page 104

top: Miles Aldrige for *Vibe*

center: Barron Claiborne for *Essence*

bottom: Matthew Jordan Smith for *Essence*

page 105: Matthew Jordan Smith for *Essence*

page 106

top: Matthew Jordan Smith for *Essence*

center: Elisabeth Novick for *Elle*

bottom: Patrick Demarchelier, courtesy Revlon

page 107: Patrick Demarchelier, courtesy Revlon

(CONTINUED ON PAGE 157)

page 108

top: Timothy White for *Esquire*

center: © 1992 George Holz for *Vibe*

bottom: Timothy White for *American Photo*

page 109: Hiromasa for British *Marie Claire*

page 110

top: Matthew Jordan Smith for *Essence*

center: Matthew Jordan Smith for *Signature Bride*

bottom: Michael Thompson, courtesy Iman
Cosmetics

page 111: Francesco Scavullo for South African
Cosmopolitan, courtesy Hearst Corporation

page 112: Matthew Jordan Smith for *Essence*

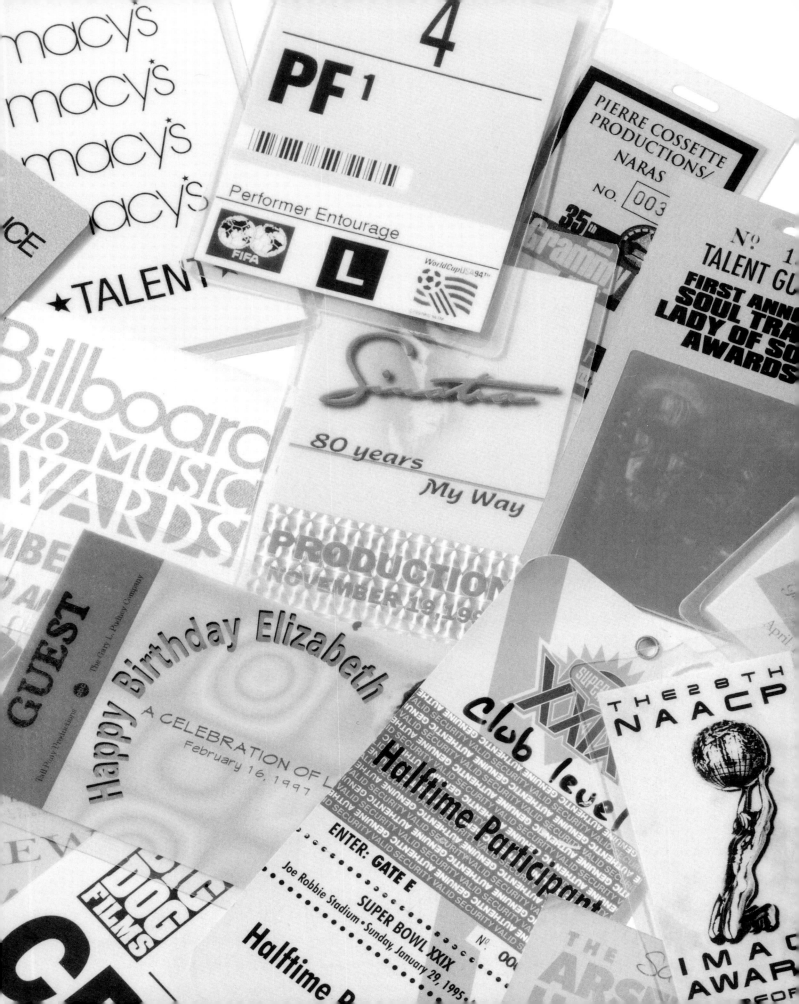

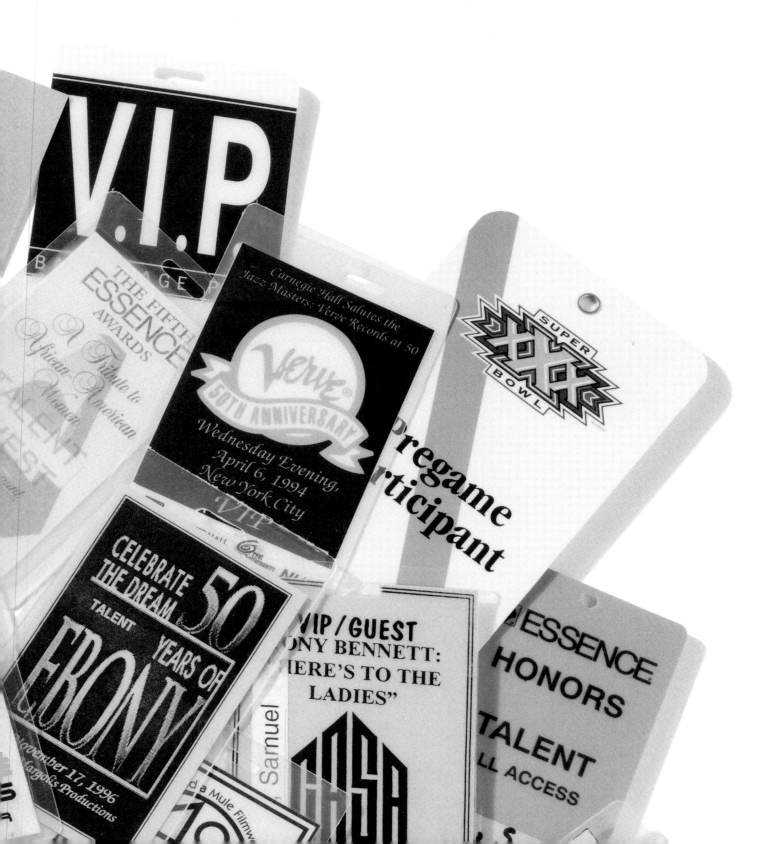

APR   1998